C-Reel Results
12 Weeks to Permanent Fat Loss and Weight Management

John Henry Creel

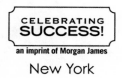

CELEBRATING
SUCCESS!
an imprint of Morgan James

New York

C-Reel Results

John Henry Creel

First published 2008

Editor: Laura T. Leggett
Photographer: Al Fuchs
Graphic Designer: Rick Shaffer, rshaffer@shafferdesign.com

ISBN: 978-1-60037-317-6

Published by:

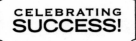 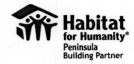

AKRIS LLC
Imprint of Morgan James Publishing
1225 Franklin Avenue
Garden City, New York 11530
330.990.0788
ron@akris.net

Dedication

I dedicate this book to everyone, male and female, young and old, who thinks they are a "victim" of the way they look and feel. This book was written to motivate and empower you to change the way you look and feel about your mental and physical self.

This book will dispel the misconceptions about nutrition and fitness and empower you to make lifestyle changes that will produce a leaner, healthier and empowered "YOU."

I also dedicate this book to my members and clients of Mind & Body Fitness, Inc. Thank you for your support, patience and belief in my quest to help people improve their thinking about themselves and their potential to change their bodies through proper exercise and nutrition. Thank you for helping spread the truth about becoming firm, toned and lean for total mind and body health!

Acknowledgements

My heartfelt appreciation goes to the many people who helped make this book possible. First, I thank my parents Henry and Mary Creel, who have unconditionally supported me in everything I do.

Thank you, Dawn Saltis, my assistant, friend and confidant. Thank you, David Meyerson for creating numerous presentations and diagrams to illustrate my principles. I also thank John Parrillo and Phil Kaplan who are icons in our industry and great role models.

The staff at Men's Journal Magazine has been so good to me, referring me often and requesting content contributions to the magazine. I also thank my staff at Mind & Body Fitness—they diligently put these principles into action every day with our members and clients. Thank you, Sean Sullivan not only for being one of my staff trainers but also for helping me compile material to document my 12-week C-REEL Results program.

I credit Erin Fitzgerald for seeing the title of the book in my name and I thank Michelle Payton, my friend and established author, for sharing her ideas and expertise. Thank you, Al Fuchs, our photographer whose talent was evident even among crying babies. And thank you, Ron Finklestein of Celebrating Success, a branded imprint of Morgan James Publishing, LLC.

Finally, I sincerely thank my editor Laura Leggett for helping me and challenging me at the same time –we make a great team! Your dedication to this labor of love helped me organize my thoughts, articulate my philosophies, and get this book written and published.

Praise for C-Reel Results and John Henry Creel

One of the Top 100 Trainers in the Nation, *Men's Journal Magazine*

"After one year of practicing the process of becoming fit and losing body fat, I have now lost 35 pounds (of body fat). I've gone from a size 16 to a size 8, and reduced the amount of insulin I inject by 40 percent, which is rare in the diabetic community!"

– Liz Edgerton, Shaker Heights, Ohio

"After four weeks of following the program, I felt like fat was disappearing! My size 12 pants were falling off and I could see more and more muscle definition in my upper body. Most of the effort came in the form of nutritional information and meal preparation combined with 3-4 days of strength training and dynamic cardio activity."

– Patty Pae, Lawrenceville, New Jersey

"John Henry Creel helped me set short-term goals so my long-term goals didn't seem so unreachable. Now I eat more than I ever have, but I went from a size 6 to a size 4 and lost 13 percent body fat."

– Mary Beth Heiman, Solon, Ohio

"My body fat decreased and I maintained my muscle tone. Today, I am 7 percent body fat and fluctuate around 170 pounds. I am stronger than I've ever been. The knowledge and experience that I gained from John Henry has made me the personal trainer that I am today."

– Joe Craig, Certified Personal Trainer, Willoughby, Ohio

"Without John Henry's help, my career competing would've been over before it began. Now I eat double the calories and am still a size 2."

– Heidi Andonian, Overall Figure Champion, IBFF, Kirtland, Ohio

"John Henry was the first trainer to teach me the critical role nutrition has in both mental and physical fitness. His training gave me confidence in who I am and in the way I look."

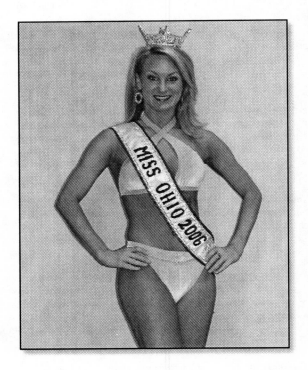

Melanie Murphy
Miss Ohio 2006, Brookpark, Ohio

"I've been dancing since I was four years old, but in five months working with John Henry, I lost 10 percent body fat ."

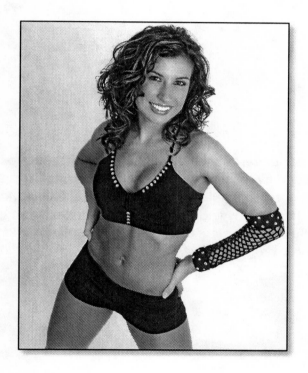

Brianne Carlon
2005-2006 Cleveland Cavalier Dancer, Kent, Ohio

Disclaimer

The information presented in this book is not intended to diagnose, treat, cure or prevent any disease. Also, the information presented in this book is not a substitute for professional medical advice. Always consult with your physician on matters concerning your medical care and treatment before undertaking any exercise and/or weight management program.

Contents

Introduction
C-REEL Results

It breaks my heart when I hear how hard many people are working, yet they continue to struggle with weight and their percentage of body fat remains high. The effort might be there but the results are not. In my opinion, people are not seeing desired results because they are aiming at the wrong target and they have simply been misinformed. They're focusing strictly on "weight loss" when there are so many other factors to consider.

To help explain what it really takes to see body-transforming results, I've come up with a program I call **C-REEL Results** – a perfectly clear roadmap to help:

- **Increase energy level**
- **Increase muscle tone**
- **Decrease excess body fat**
- **Maintain long-term results**

To achieve these objectives, my program incorporates key components that work synergistically to manifest visible results. These components are the very foundation for building a lean and slender body so I call them "cornerstones" and there are four of them.

The C-REEL Results "Four Cornerstones of Fitness"

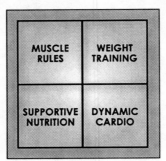

MUSCLE RULES	WEIGHT TRAINING
SUPPORTIVE NUTRITION	DYNAMIC CARDIO

Throughout chapters of this book, you'll see the Four-Cornerstone visual with one square highlighted, indicating that the information presented applies to that Cornerstone.

The foundation of my system is lean active muscle. Establishing true muscle tone breaks the vicious "yo-yo" syndrome once and for all. **C-REEL Results** is a 12-week program that's all about burning fat and improving muscle tone by developing and nurturing your metabolism for long-term results. The C-REEL Results program is presented at the end of this book –but before you jump in, we've got some things to learn.

I wrote this book because I want to be everyone's personal fitness coach! I know that's a bold statement, but I'm prepared to make it based on the results my clients have achieved and based on my passion to help people work smarter, feel better, and achieve long-term results.

Notice I said I want to be your personal "coach," not personal trainer. Personal training is part of the equation, but coaching is about EMPOWERING you with information and encouraging you to rally for your own results. To be empowered means you have confidence in your own decisions and actions. I believe that information and truthful guidance are the keys to empowering people. To me, empowerment means developing and practicing a higher level of thinking that motivates you to continuously improve the way you live your life.

I am not trying to replace your physician or your dietician, but I do share information in this book that will help you make better-informed decisions when consulting with these professionals. Any information presented here is based on personal experience, proven science and, most importantly, on long-term results my clients have achieved. You can get short-term results from many diet and exercise plans but they are usually just that: short-term.

"Bench Pressing" Multiple Sclerosis

Susan Shapiro, Age 64, Shaker Heights, Ohio

"I am almost 64 years old. My husband Paul and I have been married for 42 years. We have four terrific children and soon we will have eight grandchildren. These wonderful children and grandchildren are the absolute joy of my life. I am an integral part of raising my very active grandchildren and I maintain a demanding volunteer agenda. I garden from March to Thanksgiving in my own yard and in the O.S.U. demonstration gardens. I am a teacher by profession.

In my early 20s, I had infrequent episodes of exhaustion and strange pains in my legs, but I pretty much ignored them. Later, in my 20s, 30s and 40ss, I had several unusual "illnesses" that were incorrectly diagnosed as "strange" and viral. In 1990, I was very ill. After several doctors and three months later, I was diagnosed with transverse myelitis (TM). This was devastating and lasted for four years until I began to feel better. By then, I was diagnosed with osteoporosis and osteoarthritis. My endocrinologist recommended that I begin an exercise program, and I did, at the Cleveland Clinic. This was my first experience working out. In April 1998, I thought the TM had returned in a more severe form. After two MRI's, the diagnosis was multiple sclerosis (MS). I have most likely had MS since I was 20-years old.

By December of 2000, I found myself in a very weak condition. Physical therapy was failing me and the Cleveland Clinic program no longer existed. I needed to get a grasp on my life. A friend recommended that I meet with John Henry. I began to work out with John Henry Creel and could barely make it through 20 minutes. Five years later, I am keeping up with the group classes three days a week. I am stronger than ever and happy to say that I can bench press with 17.5 pound dumbbells, which is something I never would have thought I could do. I feel wonderful, and better still, I have not had a severe MS episode in a very long time. When I do have more severe symptoms, they seem to be resolved in a timely manner. I feel I am in great condition and intend to stay this way.

Thanks to John Henry and his entire staff, I am living successfully with the MS and osteoarthritis."

Chapter 1
Return to The Perfect You

You were born The Perfect You! Unfortunately, many people feel they've lost their perfection when it comes to body size, image, health and wellness. The truth is that your perfection is still there, although it may be hidden by emotions, issues, problems and excuses that manifest as excess body fat. That's right, excess fat is nothing but a pile of excuses, issues and problems that someone is not willing to deal with. I know that's a strong statement, but my experience has shown me time and again that excess body fat is only a symptom.

This may be difficult to hear, but think of a baby. Babies are perfect little bodies that have their priorities right: eat, sleep and you-know-what. Only when they take care of these things (first) do they thrive and develop physically and emotionally. Their food (breast milk or formula) is naturally a perfect mix of protein, carbohydrates, fats, vitamins, minerals and water. Their metabolism is working without obstacle. They crawl, walk and eventually run.

Of course, we were all babies at one time. So what the heck happened between then and now? My opinion is that somewhere along the way, the rules of taking care of our bodies were either not passed on or were gravely distorted. Our elders simply forgot to tell us we need to nurture ourselves continually.

I want this book to teach you laws of the body (how it really works) so you understand the rules associated with these laws. When you know how the body works, you can know how to take care of it. That said, many people think they "know" but still don't "do." That's where training of the MIND comes in. And in my system, the body always follows the mind. As you will see, the mind must come first.

Please know that you are perfect and special right at this very moment! If you don't believe me, that's because someone told you otherwise and you believed them. Think of yourself as that baby. We all start a certain way and I believe we can all finish that way!

Your 2 Greatest Powers

If you're like many middle-age people, you might be wondering what your body is doing and why it doesn't respond the way it used to. Every day clients share with me in a very sincere yet dumbfounded voice: *"John Henry, at one time I could eat whatever I wanted and drink a case of beer and chase those beers with two bags of Funyons and I wouldn't gain a pound. But then I turned 20, 25 or 30 and before I knew it my body changed. I had saddle bags, side pockets, a little pouch, an extra person, a tire, I looked like I was three-months pregnant, etc."* You get it. And you might have a similar story.

Let me explain why at some point, some of us start to gain extra weight (fat). At birth each of us inherently has two tremendous powers: Muscles and Hormones. When we're young, we take both for granted – understandably because no one tells us otherwise. Worse yet, is that we take these powers for granted when they're operating at their highest levels in terms of genetics, metabolism, self esteem, strength and energy. Often we just plain abuse our genetic or metabolic gifts (with the Funyons, for example). We neglect them and don't realize how a little nurturing while we're young could benefit us for the rest of our lives.

Your muscles are like batteries. You use them during the day and recharge them at night. We are all born with different types and sizes of batteries. Some of us are born with Size D batteries and some with Size AAA. I'm not referring to the circumference or size of the muscle tissue, but to the amount of energy/power the muscle can hold. Size D batteries hold more energy/power which means they are stronger and give off more energy. More heat energy is produced and that's how we burn calories/fat, especially at rest (hurray!). Most men have Size D and C batteries so they are less susceptible than women to storing excess body fat.

As babies, it really doesn't matter what size batteries we have because babies always follow the "metabolism ritual" of eating right and often.

And they are as physically active as possible. But when was the last time you saw a bunch of five-year-olds going for a six-mile run? At that age, energy levels are practically at a maximum. So it's ironic to consider that if the human body was really equipped physically to handle long and strenuous runs, it would be at its peak when we are four, five or six years of age (that's something to make marathon runners think about!).

If muscles are like batteries, then your hormones are like jumper cables. Muscles hold the energy and hormones "pump" the energy, or life, into the muscles (and your brain) constantly so they are always ready to be used. This explains why babies and teenagers want to be so active and eat often. By the way, this process or cycle of being active (using or expending energy) and consuming food then sleeping is what we call "having a metabolism!" Metabolism is perfectly nurtured in babies. But as we age, activity level and food processing power (quantity and quality) slows or ceases altogether. For awhile, our hormones fill the void even if we're extremely inactive and eat terribly. Then at some time –usually in our late 20s and 30s –the power of our hormones begins to wane and one by one the jumper cables are turned off, leaving the muscles to fend for themselves. But if there's little or no muscle, what's there to power our metabolism?

The good news is that even though hormone levels significantly decline as a natural part of chronologically getting older, our muscles can be trained to speed up our metabolism on their own, regardless of our age. Unfortunately, no one taught most of us how to nurture our muscles to protect the integrity of our metabolism … until now! That's what this book is all about.

Everyone on earth can recharge their batteries and get in shape. The real challenge becomes: what are you prepared to do once you learn what you need to know? If you learn the rules and understand the facts, then the excuse can only be YOU. And quite honestly, that's what I've found people fear the most. No one wants to accept they can't do something or don't possess the will to change. When you're fit and healthy, however, you embrace potential (the unknown) and you seek out the challenge. You know in your heart that it's just a matter of time before you will look and feel better.

Ladies and gentlemen, before I share with you the answers and solutions you need to win the fitness game, you need to be comfortable in your own skin! That means becoming mentally empowered and physically more desirable in your own mind.

Your Perfect Operating System

Let's compare your body to a computer's operating system. When you get a new computer, its operating system runs perfectly. But if you violate rules associated with the operating system, the computer freezes or files get corrupted which can cause all sorts of problems. The same is true with your body. It runs only one way, despite how much we try to manipulate, outsmart or re-program it. Just as a computer programmer must learn, understand and abide by the operating system's rules, you must do the same when it comes to your body. Learn the rules and understand how to apply them on a day-to-day basis to acquire the short and long-term results you desire.

I'm not talking about stringent diets and unrealistic regimens. When I say "rules" I'm referring to the cause and effect relationship between metabolic science and outcomes. What is most unfortunate, yet very prevalent, is that most people are trying to run their operating systems without knowing, or truly understanding the programming rules. You simply were never told. And because you were never told the rules, you don't even know what the outcome could be. Clients tell me all the time they want a great body. I tell them they don't even know what they're aiming for or what's possible (most are pleasantly surprised!).

You'll understand why by the end of this book, but the ONLY result you should be aiming for is *increasing and maintaining your muscle tone*. This, as you will read, drives everything else: decreased body fat, healthy weight management, etc. *Let me repeat that:* the only result you should be aiming for is increasing muscle tone. Everything else will manifest itself from there.

If I can teach you how to program the operating system, I don't have to motivate you. My experience has shown that educated people become self-motivated. Combine motivation with the right roadmap and we've got fertile ground for a total body transformation.

Your "perfect operating system" needs muscle to function optimally. I almost titled this book "Muscle Rules" because I need to emphasize the importance of muscle in this world where muscle is under-stated, under-appreciated and continually sacrificed (especially when we diet and as we get older). First, muscle is the only tissue that combats body fat so it "rules," as teenagers would say. Second, this book is meant to teach you the "rules" of muscle so you can understand how to nurture it, protect it, and use it to combat body fat. You must understand that lean "active" muscle is directly related to metabolism and fat loss.

Soon you will wonder, as I do, why much of the fitness information out there seems to be presented backwards. For one minor example, take the common phrase "Health and Fitness." The phrase should read "Fitness and Health" because as you improve your fitness level you are more likely to enhance your health. You'll be internally motivated to get more sleep, eat better foods more often, and stick with an exercise plan. Your fitness will improve and, consequently, so will your long-term health.

I also want to help you define your own purpose for embarking upon this body transformation journey. Knowing in your heart the "why" will be the glue that holds your results long term.

Muscle is the energy of life, the Driving Force in the body (the Dahli Lama, the Pied Piper of Fitness!). Do you get the point? Unfortunately, muscle is taken for granted in many fitness programs. Don't be scared of your muscle —especially you ladies. It's your savior! You'll be relieved to know that lean active muscle takes up eight times less space than fat inside the body.

I am excited for you to learn and finally understand that muscle IS your metabolism and your metabolism drives fat loss. A body with lean, toned and firm muscle is a SLENDER fat-burning operating system that will yield a fit and healthy body that looks good today and can be maintained tomorrow.

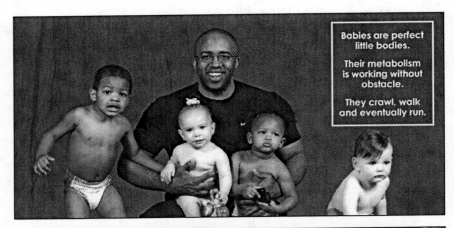

Babies are perfect little bodies.

Their metabolism is working without obstacle.

They crawl, walk and eventually run.

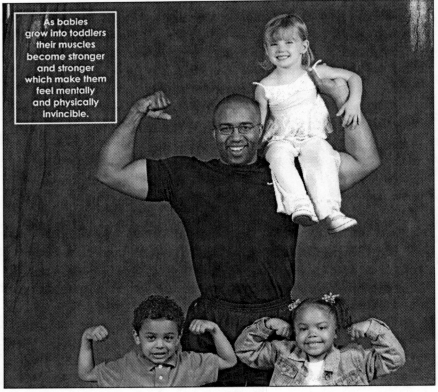

As babies grow into toddlers their muscles become stronger and stronger which make them feel mentally and physically invincible.

Figure Competitor Mom
Finds the Right Formula
Mary Beth Heiman, Age 37, Solon, Ohio

"As a wife and full-time working mother of two, prior to meeting John Henry I found it difficult to remain faithful to a strict training regime and an even more strict diet. I would start training and slack off or go on binge diets. Somehow, conflicts always kept me from staying on a training schedule. Finally, I decided competitions weren't just dreams I had for myself, they were goals. I wanted this for my life, but I didn't have the right formula to balance a strict training and diet schedule with my busy day-to-day life.

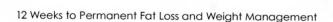

When I met John Henry, I instantly knew I had struck gold. He helped me set short-term goals so my long-term goals didn't seem so unreachable. John Henry helped me find the right balance to continue my daily life and include competition training in as well. With his help, we found the right formula of diet and exercise that would push my body to the limits I wanted. Many days, it was a struggle with the stress of daily life and a very strict diet. However, I now have the motivation to stick it out and the desire to reach my competition goals.

Now I eat more than I ever have but I went from a size 6 to a size 4 and lost 13 percent body fat. That is right! Women are scared of muscle, but, as I have learned from John Henry, it takes up less space in the body than fat. This is why I no longer worry about a number on the scale, but instead monitor my body fat percentage.

John Henry and I worked together to keep me on the path to success, toward the competition goal I had dreamt about since I was a teenager. I know I will continue training and competing. And I am now the proud mother of three!"

Chapter 2
Mind Matters

My experience has shown that fitness is so much more than conditioning the body. This book differs from other fitness books because I address the mind as much as the body. I want to help you adopt a new and healthier way of THINKING regarding:

• How you feel about yourself

• How to make necessary changes

• How to become empowered

• How to achieve physical transformation

• How to maintain a positive mental attitude for achieving permanent results

Whereas other fitness professionals focus only on building people's bodies to acquire physical results, I focus on empowering your mind so you can transform your body for a lifetime of personal happiness and satisfaction. If personal happiness and satisfaction is the "end," I guess you can say that the means I use to achieve that end happens to be health and fitness. I not only want to improve your body. I want to improve your entire self.

Let me give you a personal example of how someone helped my entire self. In this case, the means to the end was academics. As a kid I was told I had a learning disability because I was constantly failing tests and not keeping up academically with other kids in my class. Eventually I became accustomed to it and somehow internalized that I fail tests and am a very slow learner. Teachers sent me to "learning labs," which really only alienated me from my peers and enabled me to pass without having to take ownership of the process.

As a result, in college the pattern continued. When tests were presented, I became petrified of failing and often did. Finally, when I was threatened with flunking out of the business school at The University of Cincinnati, I asked a professor for help. He could've just given me assignments and told me to do them. Instead, he looked at how I thought and then explained to me that I was trying to assimilate too much information at one time. He gave me a visual formula for learning that finally worked for me. Not only did he help me graduate, more importantly, he actually cared about how I thought and gave me a feasible plan for changing my thinking and progressing long-term. Because he addressed the CAUSE instead of just the symptom, my professor empowered me and taught me how to apply myself so I could attain results in all areas of my life.

This story demonstrates with what I'm trying to do for you regarding fitness. I want to first look at how you think, then offer you a better way to acquire desired results. This higher level of thinking toward exercise and nutrition will prepare you to be a more proactive, assertive person in all areas of your life.

As your fitness coach, I'm not so interested in the way your body looks, as in the way you think about yourself and how your body works! Don't misunderstand me, a lean and healthy body will manifest itself, but only as a byproduct of the right "thinking" that leads to the right and consistent actions.

The way you think about yourself is so important. Your body responds to the attitude you have about your physical self. Quite simply, what you think about, you bring about! You need to be at peace with yourself, like yourself, and treat yourself with love, not punishment. You can't change your outside without changing your inside. Many unhappy people believe that if they can change their exterior bodies (i.e., lose weight) they'll finally be happy with themselves. The truth is the exact opposite: if they are happy with themselves, then their bodies will change. You first need to develop a positive concept of yourself.

You Are Special

You were special the day you were born, so why should now be any different? The only thing that may have gone wrong is that no one actually told you that you were special and capable of doing great things. They also didn't tell you that it was your duty to take care of yourself. You didn't know any better. So don't be so hard on yourself if you're frustrated with your current condition. You've never been given the right information or "mindset software" for your operating system.

I don't know where you come from or what you've been through, but I do know that your birthright is to feel good about yourself! The process we're embarking upon is much like how a sculptor whittles away excess material to uncover what's already there.

Let me share with you something very special that my grandmother told me several years ago. She said within all of us are several "treasure boxes" that are waiting to be opened. They're very small but contain big and valuable information that help each of us evolve, appreciate and care for ourselves and others. She said the better you are to yourself as you get older the faster each one of those treasure boxes surfaces and opens so we can use what's inside to prosper. This conversation came up because I asked my grandmother if she was afraid to die. Her answer was "no" because all her treasure boxes were open!

My grandmother cautioned me that you can't open the treasure boxes all at once because some are buried deeply and covered up by excuses, issues and problems. One of the beautiful things about getting older that unfortunately most people never realize is that you're supposed to get wiser, kinder, more forgiving, more open-minded, more proactive and less self-serving. As you get better at realizing these gifts (and it definitely takes practice), those treasure boxes will open at just the right time. I want to help you reach down and discover your treasure boxes!

Let's acknowledge your perfection that's already there and work together to paint your personal picture of fitness. The key here is "you." I want you to look and feel how "you" (and only you) should look and feel, not anyone else.

As your fitness coach, I'm here to remind you of how special you are. To ask you and encourage you to take better care of yourself, starting now! Do it for you and your family. Those you love will benefit too because you'll become a better parent, sibling, child, friend, co-worker, all the titles that make you, you!

I want you to be excited about this "meeting" between you and me. You have a lot to look forward to, and life is exciting when you have something to look forward to! Usually the unknown scares people, but in this case, let it motivate you. Neither of us knows your true potential (mental or physical). I want to help you adopt a new attitude and learn a new roadmap for mind and body fitness that you are empowered to follow.

If negative thoughts prevent you from adopting a new attitude immediately, don't worry about it for now. Just keep reading and be willing to embark upon this journey. As your fitness improves and you feel better about yourself, you'll start to appreciate the little things in life. You'll also find that it's much easier to cope with life's ups and downs. I want you to stop "surviving" life and start living and breathing it in!

Your Thinking Could Be Sabotaging You

Most people don't understand the Law of Cause and Effect when it comes to thoughts and outcomes. Thoughts are energy and your body listens. If you want something that you've never had before (a lean and slender body), you're going to have to do some things you've never done before and you're going to have to THINK in ways you've never thought before. That means being open to adopting new ideas, even if they conflict with old belief systems or "conventional wisdom."

This leads me to the number one misconception regarding health and fitness and the basis for much of what I am going to educate you on in the following chapters: Muscle vs. Fat – which weighs more? If you said muscle, you are wrong! That is the answer ten out of ten people say! There is no difference in weight between five pounds of muscle and five pounds of fat. They weigh the same! Think of the old mind teaser: which weighs more, five pounds of feathers or five pounds of steel? Again, they both weigh the same but people instinctively say the steel weighs more because it looks like it would.

Pound for pound, they weigh the same – feathers, fat, steel and muscle. The difference is five pounds of feathers takes up a lot more room than five pounds of steel. Likewise, five pounds of fat takes up a lot more space than five pounds of muscle. The FACT is that, per pound, fat takes up 8x more space in the body than muscle. This is because muscle is more dense than fat. Therefore, the same volume of muscle would weigh more than the same volume of fat. Sadly, this fact is what has misled society to think that muscle is bigger and weighs a lot. It doesn't weigh more than fat, it just has a higher density because it takes up less space in the body.

Women tell me all the time they are scared of lifting weights for fear of acquiring "bulky muscles". I hope you are now beginning to understand the truth, that it is not the muscles that are bulky, they are lean and dense. It is the fat laying over top of these beautiful muscles that is taking up all the space, making those jeans feel tight! So now I ask you, as I ask those who are afraid to perform strength training exercises for fear of getting big; which would you rather have on your rear end? Five pounds of lean, dense, and (as you'll soon learn) fat-burning muscle tissue or five pounds of bulky fat?

As you begin to understand the true differences between muscle and fat, you will begin to understand that it is not your body weight that should be your biggest concern. You should be most concerned about your body composition. When you get on the scale, you are weighing everything in your body- water, bone, fat and muscle. However, your weight does not tell you anything about your body composition, which is the percentage of body fat you are carrying around on top of those lean and firm muscles! Unfortunately, everyone is focused on their weight! As I educate, and in many cases re-educate, you on your way of thinking about muscle, you will begin to realize how it is possible that I have 150-pound female clients who wear size 4 or 6 pants and dresses. Yes, you read that correctly! This is because that 150 pounds consists of a lot more muscle, which is more dense, but a lot less body fat, therefore allowing them to fit into those coveted female sizes. Their weight is higher compared to society's norm for women, but their body composition, or percent body fat, is lower than most people's (15-18%), This is also why I have 130-pound female clients who are also wearing a size 4 or 6. The difference you ask? You better know the answer now! Their body compositions are higher! They have more fat on their bodies (25% or more) than the 150-pound women.

Now these are just a couple of examples. I have clients of all shapes and sizes. I am just comparing these two groups of women because they are wearing the same sizes. I just wanted to demonstrate to you how this could be when their weights are significantly different. Again, I'm going to restate, that people do not have a weight problem, they have a fat-management problem!

If you are still having a hard time digesting the muscle vs. fat misconception, take a look at the diagram below to see the visual difference:

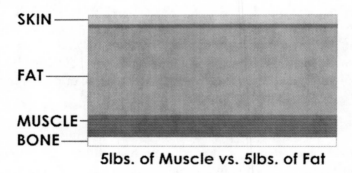

5lbs. of Muscle vs. 5lbs. of Fat

Now, tell me, regardless of your weight, which would you like to have more of on your body, muscle or fat? If you didn't answer muscle, then please go back and read the last few paragraphs! I cannot stress enough how important it is for you to understand this concept. You need to accept it and embrace it as you continue to read this book. It will help you achieve success and C-REEL RESULTS!

Unfortunately, that isn't the only fitness misconception I'm going to have you scratching your head at! Please bare with me, I'm here to teach and empower you so you have the knowledge to be lean, fit, healthy and strong! If you think that aerobic activity is the best way to lose weight or that eating fewer calories will yield a lean body, you are in store for more shocking information! You may still think that muscles are only for bodybuilders and athletes (my 88-year-old client, Betty, would beg to differ with you!). I look forward to enlightening you more in the next chapters!

So by now I hope I've gotten my point across: I care more about how you THINK than how you look! That's because I know for a fact that the body is representative of the mind. If your thinking doesn't change, your body won't change either. Think about how many people are slaves to the gym, yet their bodies seem to remain the same.

I'm so passionate about my clients having the right mindset that I strategically named my personal training studio in Beachwood, a suburb of Cleveland, Ohio, *Mind & Body Fitness*. Notice I didn't name it "John Henry's Gym" or "Muscles R Us" or even "Body & Mind." The mind must come first. And then: physical results will come, along with a whole lot more!

Personal Trainer Thought He Was in Good Shape

Joe Craig, MBF Personal Trainer, Age 32, Willoughby, Ohio

"My name is Joe Craig and I'm a personal trainer at Mind & Body Fitness (MBF). I've been working for John Henry for almost four years. Before I came to MBF, I felt that I was in pretty good shape and ate well. I thought I was eating well and exercising correctly. I had just finished my certification for personal training and thought I was finished with school. Little did I know it was just beginning.

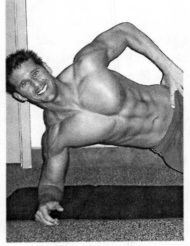

My first day working for John Henry was a little overwhelming. He had me change into workout clothes and wanted me to perform various exercises. Along the way, John Henry would stop me, correct my form, and explain why he did this. It all made sense. Over the weeks and months that followed, the knowledge and experience I gained was priceless. My confidence grew as well.

Everyone who knows John Henry will tell you they get an earful about nutrition. I thought I was eating well but I was wrong. John Henry made me realize I wasn't eating enough. I wasn't feeding my muscles the proper balance of nutrients. I also thought I was in pretty good shape. John Henry measured my body fat and I was 17.5 percent and 182 pounds. I was just above the body fat range for an athletic male. This was pretty depressing to me because of what I previously thought.

Over the next four months, I followed his guidance. I was lifting and eating the way I was instructed. My body began to transform. At the end of these four months, my body fat went down and I maintained my muscle tone. Today, I am 7 percent body fat and fluctuate around 170 pounds. I am stronger than I've ever been.

The knowledge and experience that I gained from John Henry made me the personal trainer that I am today. I lead by example. I am more confident than ever in my abilities and truly enjoy being a part of the MBF team."

Chapter 3
Empowering You

First, let's address the big picture: your thinking about life in general and your existence on this planet. For example, there's a difference between someone "aging" versus "evolving."

Stop Aging and Start Evolving

Every day I hear people put a negative focus on age, complaining about "getting older." So of course it makes sense that people are unmotivated about life in general, much less their own fitness and health. "Evolving" on the other hand means you are practicing specific strategies and tactics every day that will help you mentally grow, physically prosper and become the ultimate YOU. Read that again. Doesn't it feel good to now have something to look forward to?

So many people define themselves by age and weight. What a shame to let a number define who you are, what you can accomplish, or what you can change about yourself. Most people allow circumstances to define them. That's because they fear defining themselves. So if you're focused on age, what are you really afraid of? Are you afraid of becoming a "lesser" person? Are you afraid of failure? Of dying?

Bottom line: STOP allowing fear to control you. START figuring out how to evolve as a person! If you sit in the back of the bus too long, you start believing that's where you're supposed to be, even when the front seat is wide open! If you have average thinking, you're going to get average results. The body always follows the mind. The truth about exercise and nutrition is they are teaching tools to help you evolve into a better person as life goes on. That's what it's really all about! Exercise and nutrition cannot fill empty voids in your life. It's your job to fill those voids if they're there.

Please understand that I'm not trying to make you a fitness fanatic or put expectations on you that you have to continually maintain for life. My job is to teach you the rules. Then you can play the game to a level that fits you comfortably while giving you freedom to also live other aspects of your life. I want you to develop an exercise and nutrition plan that parallels your own personal expectations. At the very least, my program will help you develop an above-average physique while giving you the opportunity to develop a model-like physique if you want to take it a bit further.

Your Priority List

Before we can get to work on your muscles, let's take a quick inventory of your daily priority list. Take a moment and rank your daily priorities, No. 1 being the highest, No. 10 being the lowest.

Priority # 1: _____

Priority # 2: _____

Priority # 3: _____

Priority # 4: _____

Priority # 5: _____

Priority # 6: _____

Priority # 7: _____

Priority # 8: _____

Priority # 9: _____

Priority # 10: _____

Now, where do you fall on this list? Forgive me for being blunt, but for you to experience success in any program you need to "give a damn about yourself." You can say that you care about yourself, but do you really? Where do you rank in the list above? I need you to be in at least one of the top three positions. That means you must come first. I know that sounds selfish, but here's a secret: when you put yourself higher on the list, you'll be more productive and available for other priorities and people in your life. Plus you'll feel better, look better, think better, and be more motivated to stay in shape and mentally sharp.

Your Excuses

If you're not in one of those top three positions, why not? List your excuses here.

Excuse # 1: _____

Excuse # 2: _____

Excuse # 3: _____

Excuse # 4: _____

Excuse # 5: _____

Yes, the reasons behind your priority rankings really are just excuses. Of course they feel like valid reasons and some are very admirable. But let's get honest and understand that they're really just excuses. Who wouldn't want to look and feel their best all the time?

Now let's take this process a step further. What's the real reason behind your excuses? My experience has shown that often the real problem is lack of self-esteem or some emotional or mental block (and one seems to lead to the other). Usually that mental block in all of us is plain old fear. For example, you may think you're fat and unattractive, but the underlying problem is that you fear being alone in life. Some people fear intimacy and they build walls of fat to protect themselves. Others fear failure or success. And the rest of you are just being plain lazy. Sure I can be pretty blunt sometimes–not to hurt your feelings, but to encourage you to be very honest and take this stuff seriously.

Let's get whatever mental blocks you have out of the way. Take a minute here and write down some of your current beliefs about your body and the way you look and feel. I want you to be brutally honest with yourself. Remember this is your book and you don't have to share what you write here with anyone else.

_____

_____

_____

_____

_____

_____

_____

OK, for now put these excuses and your beliefs aside. I didn't say we won't deal with these issues because we will. But for now, put them aside. You'll soon realize that a focused mind and a body empowered physically is much better equipped to manage emotionally and mentally challenging beliefs.

Permission to Win

We all have life scenarios. It's easy to lose focus, lose drive and stop believing. If you don't think highly of yourself right now, somewhere along the way, you've stopped believing. I don't know what you're going through or thinking about while you're reading this book. I don't know who you are personally. I'm not even sure where you want to go. All I know is that when you make up your mind, I believe you can go and do and achieve anything you want. No matter what, I believe in you and I'm giving you permission to win. That's exactly what my college professor did for me. He didn't know me from Adam but he cared, listened and shared with me, and I've been winning ever since.

Let's focus on transforming your mind and body into a lean fat-burning operating system. In the process, I promise you'll become a more productive person, a better spouse, a better employee and/or a better parent or child.

My Part, Your Part

My part as your personal fitness coach is to explain exactly how things work and provide a roadmap that leverages the rules of our human operating systems. Your part is to believe in yourself, step up to the plate, and do something!

In the next chapters, I will explain the metabolic process. You'll understand the "why" and "how" so you can eliminate misconceptions and negative thoughts about nutrition and fitness.

At the end of this book, I lay out my **C-REEL Results** program and allow you to take action. All workouts presented will exercise your muscles and protect your joints. Don't worry, I am going to assume you have knee, back, shoulder and elbow problems because many people do. I also want to improve your flexibility and range of motion while I help you return to the Superwoman or Superman you were born as.

Prioritize, Re-Organize and Schedule

Other books will tell you to set goals and plan strategies to lose weight. You won't read that here. I want you to get out of the desperation mode that emphasizes weight loss. Desperation is fertile ground for making bad decisions (like going on a starvation diet). Instead, I want you to methodically plan your fitness goals by prioritizing, re-organizing and scheduling to accommodate your fitness. Here's what I mean:

- *Prioritize*: You need to learn to make yourself a priority and clear up misconceptions and negative thoughts about yourself and how your body works in relation to fitness.

- *Re-organize*: You need to re-organize your lifestyle so you can properly program your operating system.

- *Schedule*: You need to take action by scheduling what you need to do on a day-to-day, week-to-week, month-to-month basis to acquire the results you desire.

If you commit to doing these three things, we'll make a great team, make significant progress, and bring out the person already inside of you who looks and feels great.

Wave Goodbye to Osteoporosis!

Betsy Burlin, Age 57, Beachwood, Ohio

"About five years ago, my doctor told me I had osteoporosis and my cholesterol was way too high. As if that weren't enough, while waiting for friends in a restaurant, my husband told me, "do not wave" when he saw the skin dangling from my upper arm!

Not sure whether to send my picture into Extreme Makeover or begin a regimen of milk and calcium for the osteoporosis, a friend asked me to join her for a workout session with John Henry Creel at Mind & Body Fitness. Little did I know it would change my life.

Before meeting John Henry, I thought a diet was starving myself and exercise was endless hours on the treadmill. I couldn't have been more wrong! John Henry explained that resistance training was the key. It was just what my bones needed, my muscles would be strengthened and my body fat would decrease causing my whole look (my arms?) to improve.

So I started resistance training. While I was doing this, the nutrition plan he gave me was really a surprise. I was eating so much! I was never hungry and, over time, I actually changed my desires in eating. A great meal to me became a grilled chicken breast, crispy broccoli and a sizzling sweet potato. My favorite snacks became a protein bar or shake and I actually learned to look forward to my morning oatmeal. This was not a temporary diet, but a way I could actually live my life happily and healthy.

May 2006 marked my five year anniversary with John Henry. I am happy to say, I no longer have osteoporosis (really!) and my cholesterol is below 200. My arms look pretty good to me (my husband says I can wave again) and when my daughter got married the dress I wore was a size two and pretty sexy for a 57 year-old mother of the bride!

I also have more energy, less stress and a whole new outlook on my life. Every week I am still learning new things and do new things that I never thought I could. Thank you John Henry! My training with you will always be a great part of my life."

Chapter 4
You are <u>Not</u> a Victim of Your Metabolism!

For 18 yrs I've heard people say "John Henry, my metabolism is slow." The question itself tells me that most people don't understand what metabolism is or how it works. The truth is that people feel victimized by a slowing metabolism because muscle loss occurs naturally as you get older. And muscle is the most metabolically-active tissue in your body. So loss of muscle results in a slower metabolism and lessens your body's ability to burn calories at rest.

Unfortunately, most people think they are exercising and dieting to boost metabolism. But in reality, they are doing the exact opposite and are more flabby and weaker

> **Muscle is capable of converting (burning) fat into energy at rest**

for it. It's imperative to understand that to make a positive change (whether fat loss or muscle gain), your body requires a certain combination of metabolic expenditure and caloric consumption for that change to occur.

Weight is Not the Problem

Weight seems to be America's most common battle, but no one really understands what they're fighting. There's so much inaccurate

> **Weight is NOT the problem!**

information out there about weight loss and body shaping—people are simply confused. I believe that confusion comes from our country's erroneous emphasis on weight management.

Let me be perhaps the first to tell you the truth: *weight is absolutely <u>not</u> the problem!* Excess body fat is the problem. And our focus on weight needs to shift toward a

> **Overweight people are more accurately "over-fat."**

focus on ideal body composition. Overweight people are more accurately "over-fat" because the fat *composition* of their body is too high and disproportionate to muscle composition (lean body mass).

When we look unhappily into the mirror or when our clothes don't fit, it's not because our bones are too big or our muscles are too large. It's because there's too much fat covering up the beauty of our body, covering our muscles and their underlying tone.

It is critically important for you to remember that this is NOT a book about weight loss, although my clients' bodies do shrink. Instead, it's about achieving an appropriate body composition by developing lean body mass that positively impacts your metabolism.

The Fat Problem

When "specialists" talk about weight loss, they are ignoring the real problem — fat. To prove to you fat – not weight – is the problem let's define body composition

> **Body Composition is the sum of bones, water, muscle and fat.**

(what people inaccurately term "weight"). Most people focus on weight without really knowing what that number means. Body composition is the sum of bones, water, muscle and fat.

Instead of focusing on your weight, you must focus on your body composition and aim to reduce the "fat" component. Healthy body fat percentages for men and women are 8 percent to 16 percent and 16 percent to 24 percent respectively.

> **Health body fat composition**
>
> **Men = 8% to 16%**
> **Women = 16% to 24%**

We certainly don't want to lose bone, water or muscle. So the truth about weight management is really "fat-loss management." Weight loss leads to a skinny and flabby body. Fat loss leads to a lean and slender body.

How Should You Assess Your Body Weight?

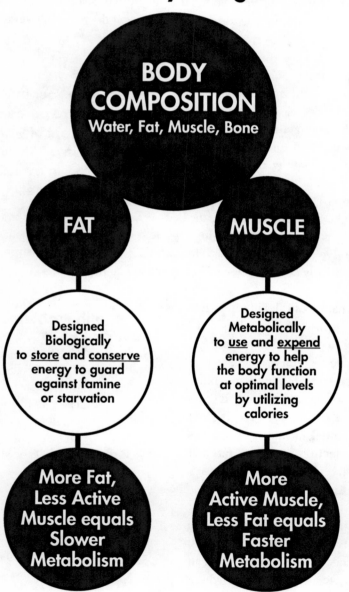

To better illustrate my point, consider the individual consequences of losing each part of your body composition ("weight"). **Losing bone** could cause osteoporosis. **Losing water** could cause dehydration. Most people don't know that depriving yourself of even five percent to six percent of water could result in a 25 percent to 30 percent decrease in overall energy level.

Losing muscle could result in loss of strength and could adversely affect your bones. Muscle protects your bones, acting as "shock absorbers." People who lack muscle risk having osteoporosis, joint problems, arthritis and tendonitis. However, in the context of weight or fat management, the most critical problem with losing muscle is decreased metabolism. Muscle is an active metabolic tissue which means it's capable of burning calories at rest. So any consequence of losing muscle is negative.

> Depriving your body of even five percent to six percent of water could result in a 25% to 30% decrease in overall energy level.

But what about losing the last component of weight—fat? **Losing fat** only makes us less fat! No adverse consequences. Yes we need some fat, but I'm talking about losing excess fat. Excess body fat is "storage" fat. It's not the essential fat that pads organs for protection, but the fat just under the skin that we're always trying to shed.

High body fat composition can lead to multitudes of health problems. Excess body fat can precipitate hypertension, which

Health Problems Associated with Being Over-Fat:
Abdominal Hernias
Arthritis
Cancers
Diabetes
Flat Fee
Gall Bladder Disease
Gout
Heart Disease
Liver Malfunctions
Pregnancy/surgery complications
Respiratory Difficulty
Varicose Veins

increases the risk of stroke. Fat can also increase the likelihood of diabetes in genetically susceptible people and bring on associated effects. Excess body fat (especially in the central abdominal area) increases the risk of heart disease. Other physical conditions associated with being over-fat include abdominal hernias, some cancers, varicose veins, gout, gall bladder disease, arthritis, respiratory problems, liver malfunctions, complications in pregnancy and surgery, and even flat feet.

When your body's fat composition is high, storage fat cells are enlarged and filled with fat. If you gain 50 pounds or more, fat cells start to multiply and remain for life. You can gain fat cells, but you cannot lose fat cells — you can only shrink them. Fat cells fight to maintain their stores of fat even when you go on a diet. Ever notice that you experience more hunger when you're on a diet? That's your fat cells fighting for survival and taking energy from muscles and organs. Your body signals hunger because it needs extra fuel (natural sugar and sufficient calories) for muscles and organs.

So if we can define the problem, why is it so darn difficult to solve it (shed fat)? The answer is simple: traditional weight loss methods make the body think it's dying so it stores fat for survival energy.

> **The body stores fat for survival energy. It's trying to protect you from starving to death!**

Your body is actually trying to protect you from starving to death!

Unfortunately, people step on the scale every day to measure weight. But, if you don't like the number on the scale, you don't have a weight problem; you have a body composition issue. Or, alternatively, my experience has shown that some people have a body image dilemma. If your issue is body composition, then your ratio of fat to muscle is too high. If you have a body image dilemma, then the way you think about proper exercise and good nutrition is not in balance. If either (or both) of these issues applies to you, take a deep breath, keep reading and we'll continue walking together on this mind and body fitness journey.

Again I need to make clear that this book is NOT about weight loss or weight gain, for that matter. In fact those who want to "gain weight" must go through the same process as those who want to lose. Both types of people must increase their metabolism. Read that again because I know it sounds counter-intuitive. Here's the difference between the two types of people: the person wanting to lose excess

> **People who want to gain weight must increase their metabolism as much as those who need to lose!**

body fat must increase his metabolism to burn excess body fat. The person wanting to increase the number on the scale must increase his metabolism to build muscle mass. Theoretically, people will fall somewhere in the middle.

The Fat-Loss Sabotage Cycle

You'll often hear experts comment on what they call the "diet dilemma." In my mind there is no "dilemma" because all diets sabotage body transformation. But I usually have to elaborate on this statement because people are so brainwashed by our culture's problematic focus on weight loss. Let's look at what truly happens to your body when you diet:

- Energy levels decrease (low blood sugar)

- Body starts storing fat because it perceives starvation (survival mode)

- Body starts sacrificing muscle (attempt to conserve energy due to lack of calories)

- Food cravings occur (attempt to restore blood sugar levels)

My definition of metabolism is the energy needed and *additional energy* required by muscles to convert food/nutrients/calories into energy and help combat excess body fat storage. You need energy to change your body shape, tone and become lean. When people diet, they restrict calories, which *decreases* energy levels—the exact opposite of what defines a healthy metabolism!

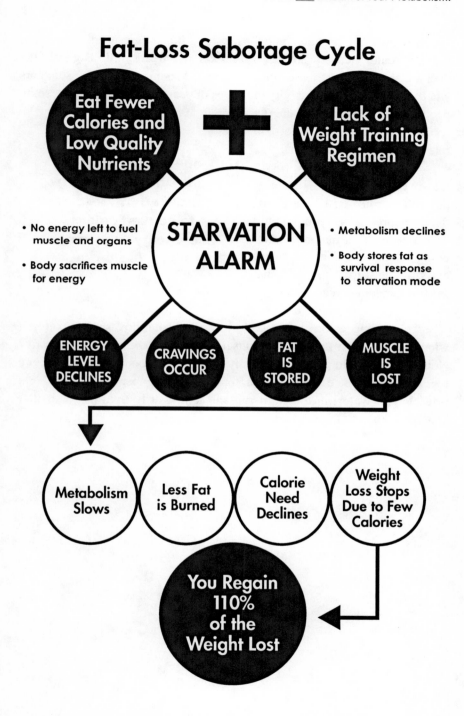

Fat-Loss Sabotage Cycle

When people are in "diet mode" they also think they need to increase cardiovascular activity so they jump on the tread mill. Big mistake because this also decreases energy levels. When I ask in my seminars whether cardiovascular activity increases or decreases energy levels, some people tell me it increases energy (probably because the endorphin release makes us feel better).

However, if energy increases through cardiovascular activity, then theoretically you should be ready to run a marathon after doing that one-hour aerobics class. So the correct answer is that cardiovascular decreases energy.

> **Metabolism =
> the energy needed
> and additional energy
> required by muscles
> to convert calories
> into energy and combat
> body fat storage.**

After restricting calories and performing only cardiovascular exercise, what energy is left to fuel your muscle, boost metabolism and burn fat? Nothing. So nothing happens to truly change your body's shape or more specifically enhance your muscle tone. A dieting person loses weight (muscle and water) in the short-run and temporarily becomes a smaller "fat" person.

What Can You Do For Your Muscles

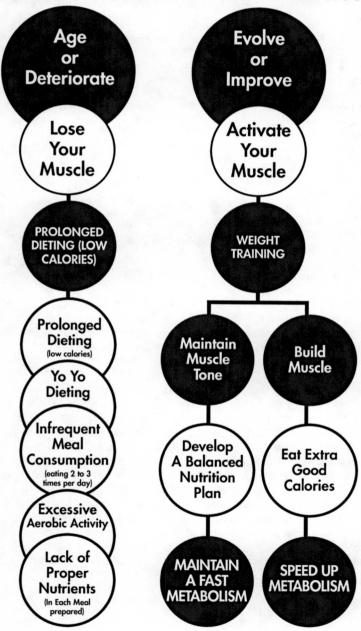

40 percent Less Insulin for This Diabetic

Liz Edgerton, Age 43, Shaker Heights, Ohio

"I am a 43 year-old Type 1 Diabetic and mother of three children ages 14, 16 and 9. I was diagnosed with gestational diabetes during my second pregnancy and became a juvenile diabetic after delivery. I have been completely dependent on either multiple daily injections of insulin or insulin pumps for the past 14 years.

After my third child was born, I gained 40 pounds due to depression and poor eating habits. This made it impossible to control the diabetes and my mental and physical health suffered tremendously.

One year ago, I walked into Mind & Body Fitness and little did I know my life was about to change in very positive ways. I began training with John Henry. In the months that followed, he taught me that fat loss and getting fit is a process that begins with focusing on your muscles, not just through weight training but also eating. After I was effectively using the weights in my workouts, John Henry and I started talking about nutrition. I committed to practicing good nutrition at least one or two days per week and was eventually ready to commit to a nutrition plan that required eating more protein, good carbohydrates, veggies and lots of water seven days a week.

After one year of practicing the process of becoming fit and losing body fat, I have now lost 35 pounds (of body fat) and weigh 145 pounds. I've gone from a size 16 to a size eight and reduced the amount of insulin I inject by 40 percent, which is rare in the diabetic community!

Furthermore, I no longer suffer from the dramatic highs and lows in my blood sugar that zapped my energy and fueled my appetite and depression. I doubt I would ever have achieved my current level of fitness without the education and coaching I have received from John Henry. My metabolism is now running very efficiently, my diabetes is in better control, and losing body fat and maintaining that loss has never been so easy!

Young and Healthy
Katie Evaristo, Age 25, Painesville, Ohio

"I wasn't eating right or exercising regularly. My excuse was always not having time and I felt I got enough exercise running around doing my daily activities. I never realized how weak my muscles were until I started working with John Henry.

I currently work out four to five days in a combination of weight training and cardiovascular activity. I prefer weights over cardio but I've realized

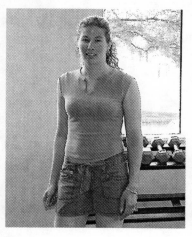

how doing a little cardio each day has made a difference for me.

Now I actually know the difference between good and bad foods. My body is extremely strong. And I hope I've started taking care of myself early enough in life to prevent the risk of disease. Today I'm doing my best to stay healthy at 25 years old, 5'8" and 130 pounds."

Chapter 5
Eating to Win

My introduction to the fitness industry was as a customer service representative for a private personal training center that also sold fitness equipment and supplements. It also happened to be headquarters for professional body builders in the area. I had always been an athlete and considered myself in pretty good shape, albeit a far cry from these body builders! Being competitive by nature, I asked the owner to teach me more about body building.

The first thing he taught me had nothing to do with muscles (so I thought). My first lessons were on proper food selection and meal frequency. There I adopted my No. 1 philosophy toward enhancing one's fitness: eat to workout and nurture muscle. I was told that all lean people (those with moderately low body fat percentage) who have high energy levels eat good foods frequently throughout the day. That's when I identified four categories of people in relation to fitness and nutrition, and they still hold true today. Most of us are a blend of these "personalities," but usually fall primarily into one or two of them.

Activity Level	Nutrition Mentality
The Couch Potato	"Live to Eat"
The Busy Bee	"Eat to Live"
The Exercise Junkie	"Workout to Eat"
The Lean-Mean Fighting Machine	"Eat to Workout"

The Couch Potato

The couch potato **lives to eat**. Food and nutrition are purely means of emotional comfort. In their eyes, all foods are equal, good or bad. If they have any concern about fitness and health, they'll diet later. They don't have any motivation to get fit and healthy unless the doctor informs them of a life threatening situation. Yet even then, because being fat and out of shape completely defines Couch Potatoes in their own eyes, things still may not change.

Couch Potatoes usually have no practical experience with fitness and nutrition, which may not be their fault. They most likely weren't raised around an active lifestyle or given any nutritional advice. Exercise is really non-existent and food becomes a haven (an escape). These people are usually eating one to two and a half times per day. They have no real consciousness of when they're eating, how much their eating, or what they're eating. They exercise inconsistently, perhaps on a yearly basis (i.e., infrequently for a year, but then take two years off).

The Busy Bee

The Busy Bee is always too busy. They just **eat to live**. They have more awareness than a Couch Potato, but they let their lifestyle and social habits dictate their nutritional habits. They are very conscious of exercise but it's infrequent, perhaps on a monthly basis (every month is different).

Busy Bees could have one or three weeks when their habits with nutrition and fitness are decent, or one or three weeks when healthy habits aren't even a thought. Busy Bees always have excuses; they're too busy, of course! They are aware and educated that exercise, nutrition and eating habits are important, but they let everything in life take priority over taking care of themselves. Busy Bees do make decent food choices, just very sporadic.

The Exercise Junkie

The Exercise Junkie **works out to eat**. These individuals usually have strong athletic backgrounds where they may have played sports in high school or college, or they were born with athleticism but never used it competitively. At some time in their life exercise becomes the No. 1 priority. They understand that being fit and healthy is important. And they know what it feels like to feel fit versus not fit. They have convinced themselves that exercise (primarily cardiovascular) is a priority and they take a systematic approach week to week. They have a schedule and they follow it. Nothing comes between them and their exercise!

If Exercise Junkies ever feel "yuck" or "fat," they are quick to add even more exercise to their schedule. Exercise is how they manage their weight and they believe you should exercise more and eat less. Or if you eat more, you should definitely exercise more. Their nutritional understanding is better than the Busy Bee's but Exercise Junkies still lack the consistency of good nutritional habits on a weekly basis. Whereas the Busy Bee eats inconsistently on a monthly basis and the Couch Potato on a yearly basis, the Exercise Junky eats inconsistently on a weekly basis (they can have one good week and one bad week).

Exercise Junkies have the best intentions because they know that activity can change their body. They are addicted to **burning calories** (yet without the knowledge of how to properly do so to achieve intended results). They are burning merely sugar; whereas they need to be burning fat. So even though Exercise Junkies are consistent with their workouts, they never really achieve results. They can't figure out why but they don't know what else to do except to keep exercising.

Addiction to endorphins makes exercise monopolize an Exercise Junkie's life and, in time, it may even jeopardize their health. The aches and pains all over are purely the result of exercise. Exercise has become religion and Exercise Junkies can't see life without it, despite not seeing greater muscle tone and lower body fat composition. In fact, an Exercise Junkie could be a size 4 but still be tremendously flabby and un-toned. The sad part of this situation is they get into a cycle where they have to work out that much more to maintain the size 4.

Exercise Junkies' primary form of exercise is cardiovascular activity such as running, aerobics or biking but they may also weight train or do yoga and Pilates. They eat rather consistently but often complain of being addicted to sugar.

Basically, Exercise Junkies have the same mentality as anorexics and bulimics. They are addicted to the thought of burning calories because they think they're fat.

What do the Couch Potato, Busy Bee and Exercise Junkie all have in common? They lack the ability to acquire long-term fat/weight management due to their under-appreciation of muscle development and supportive nutrition.

Lean Mean Fighting Machine

Lean Mean Fighting Machines understand the value of muscle in the fat burning process so they **eat to workout**. They have a systematic approach to how they exercise and eat on a regular basis. On the fitness side, they have an appreciation for all forms of exercise and they create a balance. No form of exercise outweighs another except for weight training. Everything else complements weight training but they may bike ride one day and take an aerobics class another.

Lean Mean Fighting Machines have scheduled times when they work out but things change, such as intensity, repetitions or weight so they continually challenge their body yet allow it to recover. For example, they may weight train on Monday, do cardiovascular and stretching on Tuesday, then rest on Wednesday to let the body rejuvenate itself. They repeat the process on Thursday and Friday, then take the whole weekend off to recharge. The next week they may weight train four consecutive days, exercising different body parts each day. Then take two days off to get ready for another regimen the next week. Lean Mean Fighting Machines are always trying to create a challenge but never straying too far from balance so mind and body don't have to overcompensate.

When it comes to nutrition, they know that food dictates the quality of their workout. So they have a systematic approach to eating five to six small meals per day. And there's definitely a difference between food types—all foods are not created equal! Lean Mean Fighting Machines definitely have an appetite, but they don't wait until they are hungry to eat. They shop and prepare foods for themselves because it's necessary to maximize their workout to eventually improve the way they feel and the way their bodies look. They're convinced that feeding their muscles is the ultimate way to burn fat throughout the day, even at rest. They want to burn calories just like everyone else, but they understand the best way to burn fat is to nurture their muscles through exercise and nutrition and let their body burn calories at rest, specifically while they're sleeping.

To achieve any sort of physical or mental self improvement, the Lean Mean Fighting Machine will NOT go on a diet. They're going to eat more quality food more often. Then they will look at scheduling workouts that complement their nutritional habits. They know that the better they eat, the better their workouts, the better their body will look and feel.

The Lean Mean Fighting Machine's focus is never on weight loss, but on body composition. They think more in terms of how they look in their birthday suit than in their clothes! And they eat to win.

Weight Training at 88-Years Young

Betty Woody, Age 88, Highland Hills, Ohio

"I am 88 years old and the proud mother of three, grandmother of six, and great-grandmother of seven.

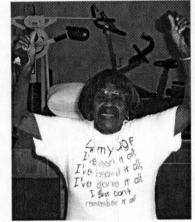

I have previously exercised doing water aerobics and walking. I have osteoarthritis in most of my joints, but I was feeling the most discomfort in my shoulders. I could not lift my arms over my head without pain. My balance had also gotten worse and I had to be careful when sitting and standing from a chair.

At the urging of my kids, I came to Mind & Body Fitness to get stronger and more flexible. Up until that summer, I hadn't lifted weights before. Within a week my shoulders barely hurt and I could lift them high over my head, which I haven't been able to do in years.

I now work out twice a week with John Henry and his staff. My sessions consist of active isolated stretching for all my joints, strength training for my arms and legs, and balance exercises so I am not as "wobbly".

It is a rare occasion that I notice my shoulders now and my balance is definitely better, too. If I can do this at my age, then anyone can!"

Come-back from Pancreatic Cancer

Sheri Grossman, Age 60, Shaker Heights, Ohio

"I will be 60 years old in a few months and am happily in the best shape of my life. I owe a great deal of my fitness to John Henry Creel and Mind & Body Fitness. In addition to giving me excellent trainers and a beautiful facility, he taught me that chocolate and ice cream are not part of the food pyramid!

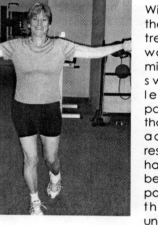

Almost three years ago, I was diagnosed with pancreatic cancer. Thank goodness I had previously started weight training with John Henry. The results have been dramatic, both physically and mentally. In December 2002, I had a very serious, delicate and complicated operation on my pancreas. The doctors told me I would be in the hospital for at least 10 days. I was home in five days and strong enough to endure the seven weeks of chemo and radiation therapies that began soon thereafter.

Within 10 days of the end of those treatments, I was walking several miles a day and swimming 20 lengths of the pool. It is doubtful that I could have achieved these results if John Henry had not helped me be in the best shape possible to handle these obviously unexpected events.

I continue my training with John Henry and his great training staff. Their attentive instruction includes weight training, flexibility and cardiovascular exercises. Equally important, they make all my training sessions fun. Their programs and dedicated energy empower me to know that staying focused and working hard will help keep me healthy and strong."

Toned and Confident

Babette Soeder, Age 46, Chesterland, Ohio

"I had previously exercised on a regular basis but was not happy with the results of my efforts—I wanted a toned body but had not accomplished it. I had belonged to several facilities previously but did not get the guidance I needed until I was introduced to Mind & Body Fitness.

I currently work out five to six days a w e e k — a combination of weight training and cardiovascular activity. I am also following the nutrition plan that J o h n H e n r y recommends. I have never been considered overweight, but my ratio of fat to muscle has significantly improved. When I started at Mind & Body Fitness, my percentage of body fat was 24 percent and it is now 15.8 percent.

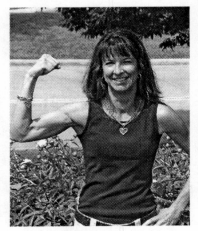

The benefits that I have experienced personally are many. I have seen a total transformation in my body. I am leaner and much more toned. I feel stronger than ever and I can do the things I enjoy without injuring myself. I find that I'm hardly ever sick and my energy level has increased significantly.

I can also eat as much as I want (the correct foods of course). A very significant benefit that is not so obvious is the stress release my workouts provide. Plus, I'm much more confident in myself."

Chapter 6
Tick Tock, Keep Your Eyes on the Clock

Mention of a "biological clock" often refers to a woman's reproductive system. But actually, both men and women have biological clocks related to metabolism. And hopefully you have a hunch by now as to why that is. Let me explain.

If you just let the body age naturally without feeding it correctly, exercising it properly, or ignoring its health on a daily basis, the body will just turn into a flabby (large or skinny) "blob" like the biological clock shown here (which happens to be frowning!). As people age or become inactive, their metabolism slows simply due to loss of muscle tissue.

The Biological Clock

I call individuals who do nothing to maintain health or muscle development "Biological Clock" people. These are the folks who could otherwise be defined as a fat-storing, sugar-craving, emotionally starving people. Pardon me for being blunt again!

"Biological Clock" people consistently sabotage their ability to get fit and stay lean. The Couch Potato, The Busy Bee and The Exercise Junkie all live lifestyles that force the body to conserve energy, storing and hoarding fat for survival purposes. Many Biological Clock people don't eat well and over-exercise to compensate for poor nutritional habits. In this scenario, they are "over-training" their mind and body and literally creating a "starvation state." They are burning up too many calories without replacing them to re-fuel, replenish or repair themselves and their muscles. And when the body perceives starvation, or is in a damaged state struggling to repair itself, three things occur:

1. Fat storage for survival

2. Illness (mental or physical)

3. Injury (or a combination of all three)

Tendencies of the "Biological Clock" syndrome are some of the following:

- They eat haphazardly, whenever they can

- They eat low quality meals infrequently and consume three to four cups of coffee per day

- They don't exercise at all but are chronic dieters or they run three to six miles per day and are yo-yo dieters

- They run three to six miles per day but eat whenever and whatever they can

The Biological Clock person has no set eating schedule and no realistic exercise approach that systematically adjusts in response to body changes. In addition, my experience has shown that Biological Clock people make many impulse and irrational decisions about their future exercise and nutritional behavior. They cannot explain what they're doing or why. As a result, Biological Clock people often complain:

- They don't feel energetic or if they do, it's only when they run

- They still have a spare tire around their mid-section

- They feel "fat"

- They exercise without results

- They eat healthy, but clothes don't fit or the number on the scale never goes down

- Their knees and lower back hurt

- Their inner thighs, triceps and back fat is "jiggly"

- They lack upper body strength

- Nothing they do seems to work

- They are too busy to exercise

- Their children take too much of their time

- They travel a lot

- They have arthritis or tendonitis

When Biological Clock people start exercising, the most popular question I get is "How long will it take me to get results?" The question represents their "temporary fix" mindset so my answer is always the same: "When you eliminate all the excuses not to get into shape." Then I explain that when they get on the right program, feel good about what they're doing, and understand why, they will start to see and feel results they have never had before. Only then will they become empowered to continue with the necessary lifestyle changes required to truly get fit and stay lean permanently.

The Metabolic Clock

So many people work hard in the gym but ignore supportive nutrition. Why is nutrition so important to body transformation? Again, it comes down to muscle. Muscle must be "fed" in a balanced and consistent manner. Erratic blood sugar levels sabotage body shaping.

When we were born, most of us were nurtured perfectly. We slept and ate consistently every few hours. We activated our muscles to roll over, crawl, walk and eventually run.

At a seminar I conducted someone asked me how I know what I know. I could've responded with my resume credentials and told her about my years of personal training experience. But when I paused to answer the question, I thought about my niece Malinda.

Babysitting her when she was three years old, I couldn't help but think back to when Malinda was an infant and I asked my sister-in-law several questions:

**Meet Baby Malinda
(now 5 years old)**

- How many times does Malinda eat in a 24-hour period?

- What does she eat and drink?

- Why does she hold my finger so tight, pull on my collar, and bounce up and down when I'm holding her?

- How often does she sleep?

**The Six Basic Nutrients:
Protein, Carbohydrates,
Fats, Vitamins,
Minerals and Water**

The answers to these questions put a smile on my face (like the one on the Metabolic Clock):

- Malinda eats every few hours or six to 10 times per day

- Malinda eats and drinks formula that's a perfect balance of protein, carbohydrates, fat, vitamins, minerals and water (by the way, these are the six basic nutrients)

- Malinda is always moving—she's flexing and developing her muscles, or in essence, weight training!

- Malinda sleeps 10 to 16 hours per day

In hearing these answers, it hit me: by describing Malinda's daily life habits, my sister-in-law just explained metabolism to me like no textbook or professor ever could! That's when I coined the term "Metabolic Clock." Think about it: at the youngest of age, we were perfectly nurtured, and — believe it or not — our exercise and sleeping habits were perfectly organized and scheduled consistently every day. Our "operating system" was not corrupted because our metabolism was unobstructed.

If a three-month-old baby eats nutrient-rich meals six times per day, sleeps 10 hours a day and rigorously uses his or her muscles, why would we as adults 20-, 30-, 60-or 70-years later, go from:

- Eating six meals per day to two to three meals per day?

- Having six nutrients in every meal to a low-carb diet?

- Getting 10 hours of sleep to (maybe) four hours?

- Using our muscles every day to near inactivity or cardiovascular-only activity?

Imagine if we let our infants live like most of us do today? These poor babies would have low energy levels, high body fat, slow metabolisms, not much strength to crawl and walk, and emotional problems due to malnourishment! Sound familiar? Keep reading because I can feel us bonding now!

In contrast to the habits of Biological Clock people, the tendencies of "Metabolic Clock" people resemble some of the following:

- They plan and schedule nutrient-dense and frequent meals

- They drink plenty of water

- They follow a consistent exercise and weight training regimen

- They go to bed at a decent hour and sleep at least eight hours per night

As a result of these habits, "metabolic clock" people often experience:

- High and balanced energy levels throughout the day

- Few, if any, food cravings

- Slender, lean bodies

- High motivation, alert, awake and ready to function as productive people

- Pain-free knees and backs

- Firm and sculpted inner thighs, triceps and backs

- Higher self esteem and confidence

- Greater ability to cope with external stress factors

- Greater ability to rebound fast from illness and injury

- More assertive and proactive

- More rational thinkers versus emotional thinkers

Unfortunately somewhere along the way, many people's lives seem to get in the way of their "Metabolic Clock." As a result, they slip into Biologic Clock habits and reap the consequences.

The difference between Biological Clock people and Metabolic Clock people is meal frequency and food quality. We need to learn how to select the right foods in the right combinations to help control blood sugar levels. Good food selection should start with breakfast, followed by small, frequent meals (approximately three to three and a half hours apart) throughout the day to help stabilize blood sugar levels.

The purpose of the Biological Clock is solely to conserve energy, storing and hoarding fat for survival purposes so the body can merely exist.
In contrast, the purpose of the Metabolic Clock is to burn and release excess fat so the body can evolve and function at its highest level (mentally and physically) on a day-to-day basis.

To increase the rate at which your body burns calories we must specifically exercise and specifically consume enough of the right calories to support a high energy level, maintain strength, and ultimately burn body fat on a day-to-day basis.

Two-Week Return from Major Surgery

Lee Handel, Age 60, Beachwood, Ohio

"My name is Lee Handel and I'll be 60 years old this month. I'm married to the lovely Amy with whom I've been with for 34 years. A better partner, I defy you to find. I have two children, Jeremy, age 28 and Gretchen, age 24.

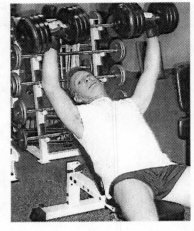

Gretchen's also a client of John Henry's and has never looked better. About five years ago, Gretchen was away for the summer. Since I'd already paid for her training, I took her place and haven't looked back since.

Up until I began working with John Henry, I'd been a runner for 20 years. Since then, I've incorporated aerobics along with weight training and nutrition and it's made a difference in everything I do. John Henry taught me that the secret is doing all these things the right way. It's the combination that's important. You can't really do it on your own!

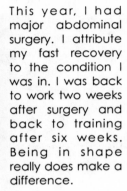

This year, I had major abdominal surgery. I attribute my fast recovery to the condition I was in. I was back to work two weeks after surgery and back to training after six weeks. Being in shape really does make a difference.

The trick is making fitness a lifestyle. I'm always amazed at how people make New Year's resolutions to get into shape, only to quit so soon after beginning. It doesn't work that way.

But if you make a commitment to stick it out for a year, you'll find you'll never go back to your previous way of living. It just becomes a way of life because you feel so much better and look better than 90 percent of your contemporaries. People tell me I don't look a day over 58."

Chapter 7
Muscle Rules

I don't know about you, but I've noticed that pretty much every circumstance in life has its ups and downs. Looking back now (I'm 39 years old), I can't help but notice that there's only one thing that has remained constant: my commitment to fitness throughout which I learned that muscle is what drives the mind and body to exist at high levels. With my knowledge of physiology, I put two and two together and concluded that muscle is, in fact, your metabolism!

From that foundation plus years of personal training, I compiled a list of "rules" that must be followed to achieve a desirable body composition that combats excess body fat.

Contrary to what some may say, rules are NOT meant to be broken! As I've said before, the body works only ONE way (like a computer's operating system). My "Muscle Rules" are fundamental, non-negotiable and based on biological science. They will help you understand how to boost your metabolism so you can combat body fat. They will also help you understand why you need to implement a weight training program, drink plenty of water, select the right foods, eat smaller meals more often, and get proper rest.

Each Muscle Rule is associated with one or more of the C-REEL Results Four Cornerstones of Fitness so you can see how everything fits together. If you remember, the Four Cornerstones of Fitness are components that work synergistically to "rev up" your metabolism so you can achieve visible results and maintain them permanently. For review, the Cornerstones are:

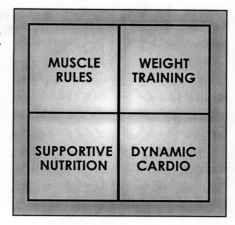

- Muscle Rules

- Weight Training

- Supportive Nutrition

- Dynamic Cardio

Following my Muscle Rules will boost your metabolism by accomplishing the following:

- **Increasing and balancing energy levels**

- **Increasing muscle tissue**

- **Decreasing body fat**

- **Maintaining results**

Rule #1: Muscle is Your Metabolism

You'll notice that the glue that holds together the Cornerstones is – you guessed it, M-U-S-C-L-E Rules! And the No. 1 rule about muscle is: Muscle is Your Metabolism!

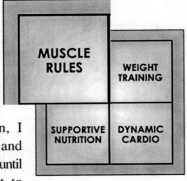

Going back to my niece Malinda again, I noticed she consistently kicked her legs and moved her arms every day consistently—until one day she rolled over! The main catalyst to this miraculous feat we all applauded was her muscle development! That's when it really hit home that muscle is your metabolism. Baby Malinda's muscle development drove her mental, physical and chemical processes to synergistically work as one unit to help her roll over.

Think of your metabolism as a coal-driven locomotive engine. The more coal you fuel the engine with, the faster the train goes. If you stop "feeding" the engine, the train slows down and eventually stops. The same is true for your metabolism. You have to "feed" your metabolism to keep it running efficiently. So it can be said that muscle is the engine that drives your metabolic system.

For every pound of active muscle you have, count on expending an extra 60 to 75 calories per day, or 1,800 to 2,250 calories per month, or 21,600 to 27,000 calories per year, all while resting. These numbers equate to up to nine pounds of body fat you can eliminate -- at rest! Did I get your attention Couch Potatoes?

Muscle is your metabolism because it literally acts as a "vacuum" or "furnace" for fat. When you activate muscle, you deplete muscle fibers of stored energy (sugar). Those muscle fibers want to be replenished and fat is a great energy "replenisher." Activating muscle "sucks" the fat toward it (which brings the skin closer to bone/muscle) so you shrink in size by getting tighter and more lean!

> **60% of cells in the body are muscle cells**

Disruptions to this process (the part most people do not address) are poor nutritional habits such as consumption of highly refined sugar and high-fat foods, and/or lack of exercise. When sugar and fattening foods are the nearest energy sources, muscle will use those before burning the stored fat we all want to shed.

Muscle is the most metabolically active tissue in your body. So when you are lean, your metabolic output will be higher. Muscular people can eat more and not gain weight because their muscles burn more energy even while at rest (sleeping). Poor muscular development, on the other hand, makes it easy for the body to store fat because there's no tissue using the energy. The amount of muscular development directly affects the level at which a person's metabolism outputs energy.

The best way to jump-start the metabolic process is to activate muscle, which is the second Muscle Rule.

Rule #2: Muscle must Be Activated

Have you ever noticed that when you pick up a baby and hold them to your chest they usually reach for and grab your earrings, shirt or fingers? Baby Malinda sure did! She was activating her muscles.

MUSCLE RULES	WEIGHT TRAINING
SUPPORTIVE NUTRITION	DYNAMIC CARDIO

In our adult world, the best way to activate and increase muscle tissue is through weight training. If muscle is your metabolism, then we want to increase muscle to increase our metabolism. If you ask me, every person over the age of 14 should weight train until they die! Is that a strong enough statement for you?

This second Muscle Rule is based on biological science, but first let me give you a personal testimonial. Weight training activated my muscles and my whole outlook on life. Until ninth grade, I was a skinny little runt and a quiet, shy kid (people who know me would say that's hard to believe, but it's true). Then in ninth grade I was introduced to and literally fell in love with weight training. It did more for my self esteem than any girl could ever do (although of course it eventually helped me with the ladies!). My body changed in ways I could not believe and I couldn't take my eyes off my muscles. I played sports and was very active in my teens, but none of that did for me what weight training did physically and more importantly personally. I wasn't a little runt anymore and I really felt good about life despite the learning disabilities I experienced during my school years.

I eventually graduated from high school and by some miracle was accepted into the business school at The University of Cincinnati where I continued to weight train four to five days a week. About that time, I started working at the personal training center. While I wasn't the brightest star in the galaxy, I was and still am a great listener. The owner of this facility taught me nearly everything I know today. I thought I was in great shape when I started there but two and a half years later with a "Mr. Cincinnati" title under my belt I left feeling and looking fantastic.

In telling you that story I may have risked losing some of you ladies because it may have sounded like weight training equates to big and bulky muscles. But get this—when I started seriously training I weighed 215 pounds and was 16 percent body fat. When I left the training facility I was 180 pounds and 8 percent body fat! So ladies and gentlemen alike, I didn't turn into the Incredible Hulk! I was a smaller, leaner and more defined fellow. I looked great in my clothes and even better in my bathing suit on the beach, not to mention my birthday suit.

Before I get into the heart of Muscle Rule #2, let me tell you what weight training did for me personally:

- It allowed me to take ownership of myself and have confidence in my capabilities

- It helped me become more assertive and not so fearful of the unknown

- It allowed me to be more proactive to achieve things I thought I could never do

So yes, weight training increased my physical abilities and helped shape my body too. But most importantly, it has and still does empower me (there's that word again) to be the best person I can be. And that's what I want for you.

So here's some of the science behind the cornerstone Weight Training and Muscle Rule #2: Muscle Must Be Activated. In simple terms, weight training activates the process necessary to transform your body into a 24-hour fat-burning machine so you can achieve shape and muscle tone. It's the only activity that provides the challenge necessary to open "little doorways" in muscle fibers called insulin receptor sites so nutrients can enter. When nutrients enter muscle cells, a few things happen:

- Energy is replenished inside the muscle so physical activity can be performed more frequently and with more ease

- Muscle tissue is repaired which leads to increased strength

- Muscle tissue becomes hydrated making it more supple, flexible and more powerful

- Nutrients are absorbed and metabolized inside the muscle tissue, making it more dense and shapely

Here is where I need to make an important point about using the scale and "weight" as an indicator of your size. As muscles receive more and more nutrients, your total body weight may increase a couple of pounds. Don't panic! Go back to the section about body composition. Increasing muscle mass is good. And if you're practicing good nutritional habits, you'll be amazed that despite a possibly higher number on the scale, your clothes fit much better. If you're weight training while not simultaneously practicing good nutritional habits, you may experience "bulk" because muscle mass increases slightly without fat loss occurring. Supportive Nutrition is the key and we'll cover that with the next few muscle rules and the third cornerstone.

Rule #3: Muscle must be Fed Specific Nutrients

Baby Malinda was nursed with a perfect balance of nutrients that drove her muscular development and metabolism. One day I took a taste of her sweet pea baby food while attempting to test the temperature. Wow, was that nasty! But to Malinda's system, it was a grand meal of "surf and turf" because it contained all six types of nutrients that were perfectly nurturing her muscles. Today the muscles in her legs are so developed that she runs around with energy and power thinking she's invincible!

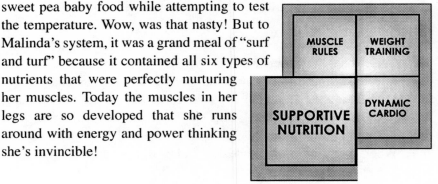

For muscle to keep your metabolic rate boosted, specific nutrients need to be consumed to balance blood sugar levels, maintain muscle integrity, and eventually help with body fat loss. This is why food selection is critically important, especially as we get older. Metabolically advantageous foods that feed muscle tissue are:

- Starchy carbohydrate sources such as whole grains

- Fibrous carbohydrate sources such as fruits and vegetables with lots of vitamins and minerals

- Lean protein sources such as fish and chicken

- Good fats such as essential fatty acids (i.e., fats like Omega 3, 6 and 9 found in salmon or some oils like flaxseed)

These nutrient sources combine to increase energy levels inside the muscle and start the accumulation of "raw materials" needed to reconstruct and regenerate structurally damaged tissues. These are the tissues that were altered during weight training. You might think that muscle is built in the gym, but actually muscle is developed outside the gym through the process of recovery which is driven by absorption of specific nutrients.

Quite simply, calories go one of two places:

1. **Nutrient-rich calories** are stored inside the muscle for energy purposes that lead to muscle toning.

2. **Non-nutrient calories** (highly refined sugar and high fat foods) are stored outside the muscle in the form of fat.

Carbohydrates in general have gotten a bad rap because of high-protein fad diets. However, the body needs carbohydrates for energy. The key is selecting the type of carbohydrates that muscle can best utilize. Muscle accepts slower metabolized carbohydrates such as whole grains (oatmeal) and fibrous vegetables (broccoli).

Highly refined carbohydrates spike energy levels and in essence "overwhelm" the muscle with unacceptable calories. Remember the vacuum? Well muscle can't "vacuum up" stored fat when its nearest energy source is lots of sugar or high-fat foods.

Protein is extremely important because it's the building block of muscle tissue and it helps slow the conversion of food into sugar. Starchy carbohydrates are slow-releasing fuel for long-lasting energy. Fibrous carbohydrates provide vitamins and minerals, but also help in slowing the conversion of food into sugar. Finally, good fats such as essential fatty acids (Omega 3, 6, and 9) allow the body to transport vitamins and minerals throughout the body and most importantly help in the fat-burning process.

These four types of foods have many more benefits of course, but for simplicity sake, I'm just giving you the basics so you can try to keep nutrition simple.

Power Foods

The right food choices give your body power—power to boost your metabolism and burn fat! Food is energy; energy is power. If you reduce calories/food, you are cutting back on your power.

People tell me every day that they are eating healthy foods, but they're not. It's not that they're lying; they are just misinformed and really believe their food selections are quality. For example, in my eyes, eating a cup of salad versus eating a cup of broccoli is totally different. The cup of broccoli will last longer and boost metabolism faster because it takes longer to digest, providing longer lasting fuel for the mind and body. For those of you who do eat four or five small meals per day of quality food and are still not happy with your results, you're probably not eating enough quality foods. Yes, you did read that right? You need to eat more Power foods at each meal to help boost your metabolism and burn that body fat! Muscle needs to be fed to have energy to burn fat.

Power Foods Nutrition Guide

Proteins

Chicken Breast
Turkey Breast
Lean Ground Turkey
Swordfish
Orange Roughy
Haddock
Salmon
Tuna
Crab
Lobster
Shrimp
Top Round Steak
Top Sirloin Steak
Lean Ground Beef
Buffalo
Lean Ham
Egg Whites
Low Fat Cottage Cheese
Protein Replacement Drink

Starchy Carbohydrates

Baked Potato
Sweet Potato
Yams
Squash
Pumpkin
Steamed Brown Rice
Steamed Wild Rice
Oatmeal
Barley
Beans
Corn
Strawberries
Melon
Apple
Orange
Fat Free Yogurt (plain)
Ezekiel Bread

Fibrous Carbs Vegetables

Broccoli
Asparagus
Lettuce
Carrots
Cauliflower
Green Beans
Green Peppers
Mushrooms
Spinach
Tomato
Peas
Brussels Sprouts
Artichoke
Cabbage
Celery
Zucchini
Cucumber
Onion

Fats (Unsaturated)

Advocades
Walnuts
Peanut Butter
Safflower Oil
Almond Butter
Flax Oil
Olive Oil
EFA's (omega 3, 6 and 9)

Guidelines

- Choose a portion of protein and carbohydrates from each column to make each meal.
- Add a serving of vegetables to at least two of your daily meals.
- Try to avoid too many simple carbohydrates such as: apples, orange juice or jam/jelly etc.
- Avoid white sugar
- Get in at least 5 meals per day. (i.e. Breakfast (Never Skip Breakfast!), AM Snack, Lunch, PM Snack and Dinner)

Powerless Foods

Simple Carbs (Sugar Based)
Refined Process Carbs (White Bread, White Pasta, Pretzels or Chips
Flour Based Pure Sugar
Cakes, cookies, candy or juices

Professional Competitor Gets Busy Living

Heidi Andonian, Age 38, Kirtland, Ohio

"I am a 38-year-old figure competitor and the proud mother of three young boys. About 16 months ago, after winning recent competition, I was introduced to John Henry Creel. The day I met him I came to his office pretty confident, bringing along photos, a detailed diet plan and a list of all the supplements I had been taking. I was there to impress. I spoke of my victories and asked him to provide a bit of guidance to help me build more muscle in my legs because the judges said that's what I needed to progress in the other competitions.

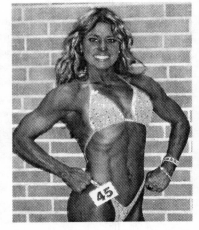

After listening to me go on and on, and giving me a once over, John Henry basically told me he had no idea how I did as well as I did or how I was even existing! I was at 1,000 calories a day for about 6 months doing 1.5 hours of cardiovascular activity five to six days a week. What I didn't realize was that I was actually doing more harm to myself than good. I was starving my body, most importantly my muscles, and there was no way I could have kept up that pace for another minute. My body was shutting down on me. I had difficulty functioning at my normal life. I'm a stay-at-home mom and

my sons were being shorted. I was exhausted all the time. My cycles stopped, I was short-tempered and worst of all, the sport I loved so much was becoming my enemy.

John Henry assessed it all and created a game plan for me. And to be totally honest, I didn't like it! I was afraid of the change. It was all new and was going against everything that I had been doing. But I had faith and believed he had my best interest in mind. When I was uncomfortable with something new, perhaps an increase in calories or less cardiovascular activity, we would talk about it. He would explain "why" and would reassure me it was all for a bigger purposes. Before, I was simply exercising and eating to compete and not to LIVE. I didn't see beyond my next contest, but John Henry did. He says "you're either getting busy living or getting busy dying." That statement finally sunk in and I realized that I was dying, or at least killing my muscles. John Henry had me do what I thought was impossible! Over time, he took my daily 1,000 calories to about 2,300 calories and reduced cardiovascular activity from one and a half hours five to six days a week to 30 to 45 minutes four to five days a week. I weight trained much more than I was used to.

I went from 104 pounds and 14 percent body fat to 120 pounds and 9 percent body fat. I had much more muscular definition and strength weighing 16 pounds more! My energy came back, I was no longer short tempered for no good reason, and I again was a well functioning woman, athlete and mother. And I still wear a size 2!

Professionally, I went from an Amateur figure competitor to a Professional Figure Competitor! In November 2006, of 61 competitors, I was named Overall Figure Champion at the Northeast Classic International Natural Bodybuilding & Fitness Federation (INBF) held.

John Henry made me understand the role food plays in our lives: why our muscles need it, what nutrients they need to burn body fat, and what could happen without proper eating and weight training. Now I'm so proud to say I'm definitely getting busy living and loving what I do!"

Power Portions

You want to eat Power Foods in Power Portions, which by my definition are perfectly balanced meals that allow you to mentally and physically "power-up" so you can optimize your thoughts and physical capabilities throughout the day. What makes a perfect meal? Each meal should contain four Power Foods: a protein source, a starchy carbohydrate, a fibrous carbohydrate (vegetable), and a good form of fat.

Supportive Nutrition is about eating the right combinations of nutrients in the right amount so you don't feel overly full, but just enough so you feel energized and strong without feeling starved.

Rule #4: Muscle must be Fed Frequently

One day when Malinda was very young her mom dropped her off for me to baby sit and I was handed what looked to me like a lifetime supply of formula. I thought she was staying with me for a week! But then my brother said, "we'll pick her up at 4 p.m. – she needs a feeding every two hours."

While Baby Malinda was getting the perfect mix of nutrients as she nursed, she certainly was fed more than three times per day. Early in her development she fed six to 10 times per day.

As adults, we too need to spread our meals out into "feedings." That may sound crazy, but once the right nutrients are consumed, then the goal is to create a consistent energy level throughout the day. To accomplish this, we need to abide by the Metabolic Clock. The cardinal rule necessary to develop a healthy metabolism is: Eat Small and Frequent Meals that Contain Quality Food in Each. I advise my clients to eat at least five (5) small meals per day, three hours apart.

Eating frequently is a fitness tool but also is an overall health enhancer because it allows your mind to better cope with stressful situations internally and externally and quickly squelch negative thoughts. Frequent meals balance blood sugar levels which directly affect your brain. When balanced, the brain is in a calm, cool and collected state to more clearly communicate with internal organs and systems.

Many people mistakenly believe they should eat less to weigh less. Nothing could be further from the truth. You must feed your muscles frequently and fuel them with sufficient calories. Eating small, frequent and nutrient-dense meals spreads out your calorie intake throughout the day which helps you burn more calories than you take in.

When you eat less food and less frequently, a few negative consequences can occur. First, fewer calories means less sugar (energy) going to your brain, which could make you tired, depressed, irritable, or all of the above. In addition, less food in your system could make you weaker because there's not enough energy being supplied to your muscles and nervous system. Worse yet is the vicious "craving cycle" that so many people fight. When blood sugar level is low, you crave high-sugar, highly refined and fatty foods. Your body is looking for a temporary "fix." You give into the craving, which is just that – temporary. You spike your blood sugar and then it drops again.

If you choose to eat nutrient-empty, calorie-less, high-fat, high sugar foods during the day (whether it be once or four times a day), pure chaos erupts inside the body. Blood sugar levels rise like a tidal wave and reach the brain with a panic signal. The brain sends a distress signal to your pancreas to release more insulin to counteract the sugar imbalance. Excess insulin is produced and your sugar level plummets due to fat storage of the excess blood sugar. While all of this is occurring inside the body, on the outside your friends, family and co-workers must beware! Irritability, depression, moodiness and impatience all occur within a 1-2 hour time period. Suddenly you find yourself saying "I'm sorry, I don't know what came over me." And so the roller coaster continues.

Infrequent or insufficient energy supply (gaps of more than three to four hours) put the body into "starvation mode" allow body fat to accumulate.

Solving the Nutritional Puzzle
Erratic Blood Sugar Level

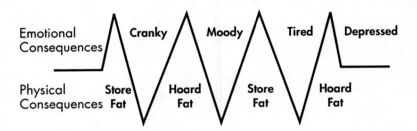

Emotional Consequences	Cranky	Moody	Tired	Depressed
Physical Consequences	Store Fat	Hoard Fat	Store Fat	Hoard Fat

Behaviors That Cause Erratic Blood Sugar Levels

- Yo-Yo Dieting
- Weight Loss Program
- Skip Meal Syndrome
- 2-3 Meal Plan
- Binge Cycle
- Unhealthy Eaters

That's because when we aren't feeding our body enough quality foods frequently, then the body STORES fat as a defense mechanism.

Rule #5: Muscle must be Hydrated

When I asked Malinda's mother what Malinda usually drinks, she told me she nurses her. Our bodies are approximately 70 percent water so that means that Malinda was getting lots of water being nursed six times per day. This would explain why children are full of energy and excitement while awake!

Muscles are 75 percent water. Hydrated muscles are more supple, flexible and powerful. You must drink plenty of water if you want your muscles to fully work for you. Muscle must be hydrated to keep energy levels high,

MUSCLE RULES	WEIGHT TRAINING
SUPPORTIVE NUTRITION	DYNAMIC CARDIO

blood circulating and all internal systems functioning at their highest levels. I challenge my clients to consume 32 oz. of water before 9 a.m. on a daily basis. Ultimately I want them to consume between 96 oz and 128 oz of water per day. Now that's a lot of physical and mental power capability! Supportive nutrition and water consumption will take practice and planning, but you can do it!

Rule #6: Muscle Requires Rest and Recovery

People jokingly say babies grow up overnight, but that's exactly what happens! At one point, Baby Malinda was sleeping 10 to 14 hours within a 24-hour period. Her development required it.

Weight Training	Supportive Nutrition	Rest
1. Damages muscle tissue so it can be rebuilt in a firm and toned manner	1. Repairs tissue to tone, tighten and shape muscle	Helps mind and body recover so in time the body reshapes into a lean, toned, and fantastic-looking fat-burning machine!
2. Depletes stored energy	2. Replenishes energy stores	

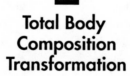

Total Body Composition Transformation

Just as Malinda's development required rest, so does ours. The toning process requires recovery and repair. Muscle contraction during weight training depletes the muscle of energy. This depletion sets up a recovery process where the muscle must regenerate and replenish itself. In short, our goal is to get the body to use fat during this recovery process.

We want the body to RELEASE fat as energy instead of storing it! **More stored fat is used in the recovery process than through any other**

activity. Please re-read and understand this last sentence because it explains the difference between weight training and other exercise activities.

The best recovery practice is rest. So be sure to get proper rest. In addition, vary your workouts to allow worked muscle groups to rest the next day.

Rule #7: Muscle must be Protected from Cardiovascular Activity

Many people might say I hate aerobic or cardiovascular exercise. That's not true. In fact, the heart is a muscle itself! But like everything you've read so far, everything has its proper role in enhancing metabolism so the body can become a viable fat-burning tool.

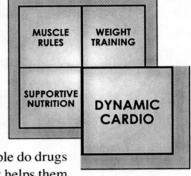

I do believe people abuse aerobic activity by using it as a primary weight management or weight-loss tool. Many people say they run because they feel better temporarily and it helps them cope with life's stressors. But be careful—people do drugs because they feel better temporarily and it helps them cope with life's stressors! That leads to addiction where the only time a drug addict feels good is when he's doing drugs. The same occurs with big-time runners. I'm being frank here because I see this problem almost every day. I tell my clients if they can't be okay without running for a week they are probably addicted to it.

Interestingly, I see runners and aerobic queens in all shapes and sizes. If aerobic activity is supposed to be the ultimate fat-burning tool, then why are runners always complaining to me about their lack of muscle tone or spare tire around their mid-sections? Many of them have terrible eating habits, too, because they are Exercise Junkies who work out to eat.

Sometimes I see people who are weight training but combining it with excessive cardiovascular activity and wondering why they're not developing any muscle tone. I tell them their bodies are using muscle as "cardio chow" meaning their marathon runs force the body to sacrifice the very muscle they're trying to build with weights.

Cardiovascular activity is a great endurance (sugar-burning) activity and stress management tool. If your goal is to run a marathon or to simply manage stress, then heavy cardiovascular activity is the answer. However, if you want a toned and lean body, then the efficiencies created by heavy cardiovascular activity actually work against you. Let me explain.

Efficiency is positive when running a business, but has the opposite effect on a workout/nutritional regimen. The more efficient your body becomes during cardiovascular activity, the fewer calories it burns (read that again!). Think of individuals who perform the same cardiovascular workout (i.e. jogging, aerobic classes) week after week. Initially, they will lose weight and experience some muscle toning. However, they eventually plateau and complain that they aren't seeing more results. They never look much different because their bodies have adapted and become so efficient performing the same activity that they no longer need to expend much energy. And here's the key: Without the need to expend much energy, calories are not required, which leads to fat gain or fat maintenance.

To force your muscles to burn fat, there needs to be a challenge that makes your muscles continually re-adapt to use energy instead of conserving it. Why do we need that challenge to burn fat and tone muscle? Challenging your muscles causes them to increase your metabolic rate by forcing your body to recover. More stored fat is used in the recovery process than through any other activity. The recovery period associated with weight training lasts 24 to 48 hours AFTER the workout! Contrast that with the recovery period associated with cardiovascular activity which lasts only one to 12 hours. This tremendous difference means that weight training has a far greater effect on resting metabolic rate (your body's ability to burn fat) than any cardiovascular activity.

I endorse what I call "Dynamic Cardio" which works to burn fat and improve your stamina in contrast to testing endurance, which will most likely sacrifice muscle. Dynamic Cardio is shorter in length and seeks to take the "efficiency" out of your run, swim or bike ride. For example, do sprint intervals instead of long and paced endurance sessions. An effective interval program should last only 15 to 20 minutes, plus a five-minute warm-up and five-minute cool down. You can perform dynamic cardiovascular workouts three to four times a week, preferably after your strength training workout when your body's glycogen (stored sugar) stores are depleted. By performing cardiovascular activity immediately after your weight workout, your body will have to use stored body fat for energy due to low glycogen levels.

You don't need to be able to run for an hour to be heart healthy. Increasing your stamina, not your endurance, is not only great for your heart but will also allow you to tone muscles and burn body fat more effectively. And you will recover faster from workout to workout.

In summary, cardiovascular activity is a great way to maintain the results achieved from weight training and supportive nutrition, when properly implemented. First, weight train; second, eat enough nutrient-rich foods; and third, perform cardiovascular activity periodically. Rest as long and as often as you need to recuperate.

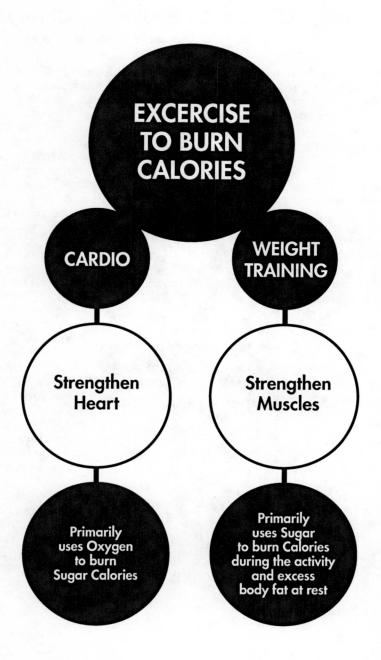

Chance Referral is Life-Changing

Patty Pae, Age 39, Lawrenceville, New Jersey

"I began working with John Henry Creel in 2001 to get back on track with my health and fitness, as I had reached a point at which I was getting no where doing it my way.

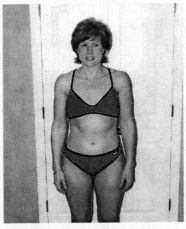

I was making things worse for me and I didn't know how to fix it. For the past eight years, I had spent the majority of my time building my career, while at the same time trying to live what I thought was a healthy, fit lifestyle. I thought I was "working out" and incorporating athletic activities and "good sensible eating habits" into my life. Well, if I was doing everything correctly why did I reach an all-time high of 164 pounds, measuring 34 percent body fat and wearing a size 12 pant?

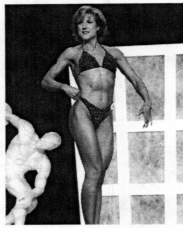

I thought to myself, "Well, that's not too bad, if I could just lose 15 pounds I should be a new person and in the best shape of my life!" Well, those results did come and, much to my surprise, faster than I could have ever expected.

Most of the effort came in the form of nutritional information and meal preparation combined with 3-4 days of strength training and dynamic cardio activity. After four weeks of following the program, I felt like fat was just disappearing from my body. My size 12 pants were falling off and I could see more and more muscle definition in my upper body.

I didn't think my strength programs were all that intense. I started to understand that it's not just the strength training that builds lean muscle, but proper nutrition, water intake, and rest are all very important too.

Never did I realize that by a chance referral to John Henry Creel, my life would be completely transformed—physically (I'm now a size 4), nutritionally and mentally."

"Muscle Lean" Cancer Survivor

Ev Carr, Age 56, Lyndhurst, Ohio

"In 2003, at age 54, I was diagnosed with breast cancer and had lumpectomy surgery that also removed lymph nodes under my arm. That was followed by six weeks of daily radiation treatments.

Before the cancer, I had been exercising, but had to stop during recovery. After surgery and radiation, I was inactive, in near constant pain and depressed. All of the medical professionals warned me I could not exercise like before, that lifting anything more than light weights risked lymphedema and/or permanent damage. I became weaker, more depressed and the surgery/radiation area continued to be stiff and painful.

Then I signed up for a weekly cancer survivor program that happened to be located next door to Mind & Body Fitness. I liked doing the exercises, but was afraid to injure the radiated area and kept remembering all the exercise warnings. John Henry's expertise, patience and enthusiasm allowed me to work safely and progress like I had not believed possible. Exercising safely, making progress and feeling better lifted my spirits and gave me back my confidence.

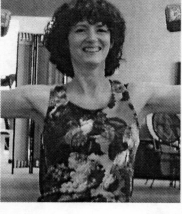

With some anxiety, I began two half-hour training sessions a week with John Henry. His passion for making me believe in myself and what I can accomplish made me dig deeper. That allowed me to continue growing stronger physically through weight training and supportive nutrition and stronger mentally through commitment and concentration. My training is now three days a week, sometimes four, far more demanding and usually one hour or more.

I was an out-of-shape size 8. Today, I am 56 years old and a size 4. I weigh 105 pounds, as I did in college, but now I am "muscle lean," in the best shape of my life, and far more confident and outgoing.

While I still have physical side effects from my bout with breast cancer, I don't focus on them anymore. John Henry and his staff continue to make a huge positive difference in my life and my outlook. I also couldn't have done this without my wonderfully supportive husband, family and friends."

Rapid Recovery from Knee Replacements

Sally Roman, Age 64, Shaker Heights, Ohio

"I have a very busy life as a wife, a mom and a grandma to Matt, Katie, and Sara. I also work full-time as a kindergarten teacher and I am 64 years old.

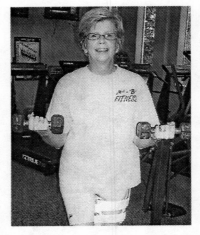

I have experienced the early onset of osteoarthritis leading to both my hips being replaced 13 years ago. This year I had to have both my knees replaced. Good nutrition and exercise, specifically weight training, have played a major role in both my preparation for successful surgery and in my rapid, strong recovery.

Weekly workouts including both weight training and cardiovascular activity helped me develop a strong body and a good attitude. With John Henry's guidance, I now understand the importance of protein and its role in building muscle. Strong muscles made the physical therapy that followed my knee replacements much easier.

Because much of the therapy was similar to the exercise routine I was accustomed to at Mind & Body Fitness, I could quickly adapt to the exercises the physical therapist had me do. I also understood how the strength training would contribute to my recovery and make my hip and knee joints more stable. Exercise has helped me maintain a positive attitude toward all aspects of my life!"

Anorexia Transformed

Stacey Hertz, Age 52, Mayfield Heights, Ohio

At a mere nine years old, I looked at myself in the mirror and decided that I was fat. At that time, my weight dropped from 73 pounds to 60 pounds and I struggled with the fear of eating thereafter.

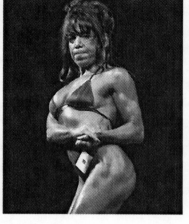

Twelve years ago, when I started training with John Henry Creel, I was anorexic, weighing 90 pounds with little muscle tone. I was a size zero, constantly injured and measured 32% body fat. I ate about 800 calories per day consisting mostly of Diet Coke and M&Ms.

During an aerobic class, a buddy of mine picked me up and actually fractured four of my ribs. I was absolutely obsessed with exercise, constant starvation and poor body image.

I bonded immediately with John Henry and knew I had found a trainer whom I could trust. He taught me to focus on building muscle to burn fat instead of starving myself, which was counterproductive. He also reduced my cardio activity from two 45-minute sessions per day six days a week to one 30-40 minute session per day four days a week.

Today, I'm still a size zero but fluctuate between a more healthy 108 and 112 pounds. I have great muscle tone and am down to 19% body fat. Instead of Diet Coke and M&Ms, I consume a total of 1,300-1,500 calories across five meals per day with variety such as chicken breast, broccoli, sweet potatoes and oatmeal. I feel and look much better! My lifestyle has transformed. I can't thank John Henry enough for all his support, care, patience, teachings and the utmost confidence in my ability to change.

What is the Real Problem?

With so many types of diets and multiple fitness options out there, why are so many people struggling to get results? There are a few answers to that question. The quick answer is FAT. The long answer is lack of understanding about muscle. Failure to lose fat is the problem. Maintaining fat loss by building muscle is the solution.

But the underlying problem is ignorance and misinformation. No one ever talks about how muscle builds metabolism and how diets destroy muscle. Without creating and activating muscle, people cannot maintain weight loss because they haven't established the metabolism necessary to support long-term health and fitness. In fact, more than 95 percent of all those who lose weight (muscle and water) following a diet gain 110 percent of the weight (in fat) back within three years!

Some professionals say diets don't work because they leave you deprived. A better answer is that diets work in the short-term because they deprive you of a lot of water. In the long-term, diets destroy muscle due to lack of caloric intake. Muscles need calories and certain nutrients to exist. 75 percent of muscle is water so if you lose muscle you lose water. Most weight loss is water and muscle. And muscle loss results in a slower metabolism. This is why most people who lose weight gain it back plus some.

Isn't Weight Loss the Answer?

First, let's understand the term "weight" (body composition). Weight is bone, water, muscle and fat. If you lose weight, you lose all four components. What are the negative consequences of losing even a little of each of these?

- A "little" bone loss could = osteoporosis

- A "little" water loss could = dehydration

- A "little" muscle loss could = loss of strength and decrease in metabolism

- A "little" fat loss = a "little" less fat!

Ah-ha! We may be on to something! The goal is to lose fat without losing the rest of your body composition.

Doesn't Muscle Weigh More than Fat?

You won't believe my answer. You really need to see it to believe it. If you take 5 pounds of muscle and compare it to 5 pounds of fat, you'll see that the fat takes up 8 times more space in the body than muscle. And both are 5 pounds! So no, muscle does not weigh more than fat.

Shouldn't I Just Eat Less to Weigh Less?

Actually, I want my clients to eat more of the right foods, more often. Contrary to common knowledge, diets destroy muscle. Under-eating also destroys muscle. I teach my clients to eat what I call "power portions." Every meal should contain the right combination of nutrients for a specific fitness purpose and in the right amount to boost metabolism. I want people to "eat to work out" versus "working out to eat." Feed your muscles and let your muscles propel your fitness and health to new levels.

Isn't Aerobic Activity the Best Way to Burn Fat and Shape Up?

Many people try to use cardiovascular activity as a weight management tool. Cardiovascular activity is first a great endurance (sugar burning) and stress management tool. For it to be the most effective as a fat burning tool, we first must weight train to build and protect our muscles. And we must EAT enough food to nurture the muscle. Then we can add on cardiovascular activity – assuming those two things are accomplished – to create the ultimate caloric deficit that we need to brush away fat.

What Should My Expectations Be?

The answer depends on what your objective is. Is your main focus to run a marathon or to burn fat? These are two different objectives and require different processes to achieve results.

Aren't Muscles Just for Body Builders?

Absolutely not. Muscle is the engine of life. It's the life-source of metabolism.

Everyone should strength train to build muscle because muscle has the ability to use or burn calories (i.e., fat) at rest, up to 48 to 72 hours later after a specific exercise has been performed. Your muscles must be activated to optimally burn calories while at rest. The most effective way to activate muscle is to weight train.

So don't let muscle scare you! It's actually your savior! By nature, men have muscle, but need to nurture it. On the other hand, ladies must create muscle and then nurture it. By nature, ladies don't have the hormonal makeup to get bulky.

Isn't Doing Something Better than Doing Nothing?

It depends on your expectation. It is not what you do that's so important as is the reason behind what you're doing. For example, are you working out to train for a marathon or is your sole purpose to build a fat-burning body? If you can answer the "why" behind your activity, then you'll know if what you're doing is driving toward the results desired. If the process supports the expectation, then you'll most likely achieve permanent results.

How Much Food Should I Eat?

There are many complex formulas to estimate what you should eat based on many variables. But to keep it simple, I ask people to tell me how many calories they are taking in each day in terms of carbohydrates, proteins and fats. If you can't tell me this, then you're most likely eating too much of the wrong types of foods. Notice I didn't say you are eating too much food, period. You're probably selecting a lot of processed foods that are empty calories. These types of foods satisfy your emotions but leave you nutritionally bankrupt. Foods that are nutritionally empty have no real metabolic purpose to help you nurture and protect your muscles. And they will not keep your energy level balanced to help combat body fat. Just as important as what you eat is when you eat, both of which have a profound effect on how your body processes the calories you feed it.

You need to make sure you can make quality food selections if not every meal, then at the majority of meals. People tell me every day that they are eating healthy, but they are not. It's not that they're lying, as they are misinformed and really think their food selections are quality. For example, in my eyes, eating a cup of salad versus eating a cup of broccoli is totally different. The cup of broccoli will last longer and boost metabolism faster.

12-Week C-REEL Results Program
Overview

The C-REEL Results program is specifically designed to re-program your metabolism so you'll see real results within 12 weeks and you'll also maintain those results.

Some of you may already be following a fitness and nutrition program that could be technically flawed or that doesn't have the proper materials, variables, intensity level or progression to challenge your metabolism. C-REEL Results will help you make adjustments so you are not wasting time or effort.

My program is set up to build weekly with exercise routines and supportive nutrition guidelines (which I call "homework). If you find yourself saying, "I already do this" or "This is too easy" and you're tempted to start at Week 6 instead of Week 1, please do NOT skip ahead! Appease me and be patient. Somewhere in those first six weeks, you're going to realize why you've been struggling all these years.

As you start the program –which is the hardest part –keep in mind some of the reasons you may have for reading this book from cover to cover:

- You are tired of feeling tired, lazy and out-of-shape

- You want to lose excess body fat

- You've been exercising consistently for years, and in the back of your mind, you're not sure if you've been doing the right thing.

- You no longer want to be a Couch Potato! Although you hate thinking about working out and eating better, if you must do something, you want a relatively pain-free program to follow that will get you results.

The secret behind my program is learning how to build your metabolism instead of destroying it as you age. We want to build your muscle tone without jeopardizing it due to improper exercise and nutritional habits. The ultimate goal is to reduce excess body fat and learn the critical role food plays in re-shaping your body from head to toe. If you need help for any reason, refer to your local fitness professional or nutritionist and let them also hold you accountable.

Do I Have to Do This Forever?

Any exercise and nutrition plan should be planned for a specific time period instead of for the rest of your life. The time-specific plan should be sound, logical and metabolically driven (here is where most people go wrong) to create results NOW. After a specific time period (in this case, 12 weeks), you should be able to combine old habits in moderation to create a realistic lifestyle that will maintain the results you worked so hard to achieve within the 12 weeks. You are not expected to eat and exercise perfectly 365 days a year. Commit to learning how to exercise smart and eat correctly to increase muscle tone and reduce excess body fat during this 12-week period. After 12 weeks, your new and improved metabolism will allow you to maintain results without feeling deprived or guilty when occasionally you might not eat so well.

For those of you who are exercise and nutrition fanatics but are not getting the results you want, your problem may be that you adhered to a strict nutritional plan too long and forced your body to adapt and become too efficient in assimilating food. Remember, efficiency is a good thing for business but not for creating a fat-burning body. When the body adapts and it's no longer challenged, it could store or hoard fat for survival purposes.

Two Programs in One

C-REEL Results is a plan for both now and later. By following the C-REEL Results program, you can construct a sound exercise program and build a productive fat-burning nutritional plan. Seeing results now will help you capture the spirit, become empowered today and be excited. Maintaining those results will help preserve your mind and body for the rest of your life.

I appreciate and commend you for embarking upon this journey and committing yourself to hard work, sacrifice and dedication. You may not follow the plan perfectly every day because none of us is perfect. But, remember, you can always return to the perfect YOU!

P.S. – There are two more things I want you to do for yourself: 1) Call or visit one of your relatives or close friends and tell them that you love them; 2) Call or visit someone you have not talked to or seen in 15 years and tell them "I was just thinking of you".

Equipment Needed for 12-Week C-Reel Results Program

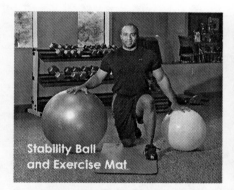

Stability Ball and Exercise Mat

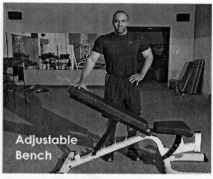

Adjustable Bench

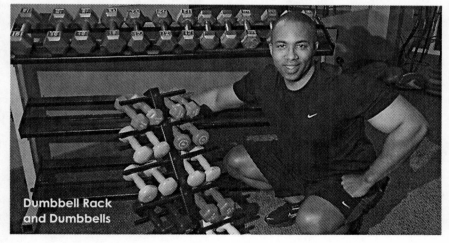

Dumbbell Rack and Dumbbells

Power Meals
Each one of these is a perfect power meal!

Option 1
1 English Muffin
2 teaspoons peanut butter
1 cup skim milk

Option 2
3 oz. Chicken breast
1 cup broccoli
Garden salad, 2 Tbsp. fat free dressing

Option 3
1 handful almonds
1 cup cottage cheese

Option 4
4 oz. turkey
1 pita – whole wheat, 7 inch
2 leaves lettuce
1 tbsp. honey mustard
1 cup strawberries

Option 5
1-2 scoops of whey protein
drink in 8 oz. water (great 4pm option)

Option 6
4 oz. Italian Grilled Chicken
1 cup salad vegetables
w/nonfat salad dressing
½ cup whole wheat pasta
1 medium peach

Option 7
½ cup blueberries
1 cup hot oatmeal
2 egg whites scrambled

Option 8
4 ounces broiled fish fillet
(w/ 3 Tbsp. cocktail sauce optional)
1 cup green beans
1 cup salad greens with 2
tablespoons salad dressing

Option 9
1 cup Multi-Grain/ non-sugar Cereal
1 grapefruit
½ cup skim milk

Option 10
4-6 egg whites w/ tossed salad
2 Tbsp. fat free dressing
w/ Choice of:
1 cup brown rice or ½ cup corn

Option 11
3 ounces tuna fish
2 rice cakes
1 cup vegetable medley
(corn, carrots, and peas)
1 medium orange

Option 12
½ cantaloupe
½ cup hot oatmeal
1 cup skim milk
2 egg whites scrambled

Option 13
4 ounces round steak
1 cup brussel sprouts

Option 14
1 Tbsp natural peanut butter
2 rice cakes

Option 15
Protein Bar w/ 16 oz. water
(great 4 pm option)
1 cup cottage cheese
½ cup of blackberries

Supportive Nutrition

Breakfast

Option 1
1 English Muffin, 2 teaspoons peanut butter, 1 cup skim milk

Option 2
½ cup blueberries cooked with 1 cup hot oatmeal, 2 egg whites, scrambled

Option 3
1 cup multi-grain/non-sugar cereal, 1 grapefruit, ½ cup skim milk

Option 4
½ cantaloupe, ½ cup hot oatmeal, 1 cup skim milk, 2 egg whites scrambled

Option 5
1 bagel – whole grain, ½ cup Cottage Cheese

Lunch

Option 1
3 oz. tuna fish, 2 rice cakes, 1 cup vegetable medley (corn, carrots, and peas), 1 medium orange

Option 2
4 ounces Italian Grilled Chicken, 1 cup salad vegetables with nonfat salad dressing, ½ cup whole wheat pasta, 1 medium peach

Option 3
Garbanzo bean/chick pea Salad, 1 medium baked sweet potato, 1 medium apple

Option 4
Tofu or Chicken stir fry (large bowl), 1 Cup salad vegetables with low fat Italian dressing

Option 5
4 oz. turkey, 1 pita – whole wheat, 7 inch, 2 leaves lettuce, 1 Tbsp. honey mustard, 1 cup strawberries

Supportive Nutrition

Mid-Morning/Mid-Afternoon Snack

Option 1
1 cup nonfat, sugar free yogurt (10am option only), ½ cup fresh strawberries or blueberries

Option 2
1 cup skim milk, 2 scoops of whey or soy protein powder

Option 3
1-2 scoops of whey protein drink in 8 oz. water (great 4pm option)

Option 4
1 Tbsp natural peanut butter, 2 rice cakes

Option 5
1 handful almonds, 1 cup cottage cheese

Option 6
1 cup cottage cheese, ½ cup of blackberries

Option 7
Protein Bar w/ 16 oz. water (great 4pm option)

Please Note:
The above options have suggested quantities. Choose a quantity that is right for you.

Starchy Carb Options

1 Large Baked Potato w/ Non-Fat Sour Cream
(10am only)

1 Cup Sugar Free Vanilla Yogurt

Supportive Nutrition

Dinner

Option 1
4 ounces Tuna Steak, 1 cup vegetable medley

Option 2
Tofu Stir Fry (large bowl), 1 cup salad vegetables, 2 Tbsp. low-fat salad dressing

Option 3
4 oz. round steak, 1 cup asparagus

Option 4
4 oz. broiled fish fillet, 1 cup green beans, 1 cup salad greens
2 Tbsp. low-fat salad dressing

Option 5
3 oz. Chicken breast, 1 cup broccoli, 1 cup salad greens
2 Tbsp. low- fat salad dressing

Option 6
4-6 egg whites w/ 2 cups tossed salad, 2 Tbsp. low-fat salad dressing

Please Note:
For each dinner option above, add one Starchy Carb option from the three listed. Remember, you must eat your carbohydrates to become lean!

The above options have suggested quantities. Choose a quantity that is right for you.

Starchy Carb Options

½ Cup of Brown Rice

Medium Sweet Potato

3 oz. to 5 oz. of Squash or Navy Beans

C-REEL RESULTS – Starter Recipes

Fruit Frostie

1 – 8 oz. container nonfat sugar free vanilla yogurt
$1/3$ cup of skim milk
$1/2$ cup frozen berries (blackberries, raspberries, or strawberries)

Place all ingredients in a blender and puree until smooth. Pour mixture into a tall glass, and eat with a spoon.

Makes 1 serving, 169 calories per serving

Curried Chicken Salad

1 package (about 1 pound) skinless chicken breasts, baked or boiled
1- 6 oz. can unsweetened pineapple juice
4 tablespoons raisins
½ cup boiling water
1 medium onion, finely chopped
1 medium carrot, grated
1 tablespoon curry powder
½ teaspoon salt
¼ teaspoon ginger
5 tablespoons nonfat, sugar-free vanilla yogurt
Romaine lettuce

In a microwave dish, pour pineapple juice over chicken. Cover and microwave on high for 1 minute. Turn pieces over and rotate dish.

Microwave for another minute. Let chicken stand 5 minutes.

In a small bowl, pour boiling water over raisins to plump them up. Set aside.

Remove chicken from dish, reserving 2 tablespoons juice. Cut chicken into bite-sized pieces, and place in a large bowl with onion and carrot. Drain raisins and add to bowl. Stir in spices, reserved pineapple juice, and yogurt. Mix well.

Chill 2 hours or longer. Serve on Romaine lettuce.

Makes 4 servings, 179 per serving

C-REEL RESULTS – Starter Recipes (continued)

Oven "Fried" Fish

4 cups Corn Chex cereal
3 egg whites
½ cup skim milk
1 pound ocean perch fillets or other white fish

Preheat oven 400 degrees. Blend cereal in a blender until fine. Transfer to a mixing bowl, and set aside.

In a small bowl, beat egg whites and skim milk until well blended. Dip fish fillets into egg mixture, then roll in cereal mixture, coating both sides.

Spray a cookie sheet several times with nonstick cooking spray. Spread fillets on cookie sheet. Lightly coat fillets with cooking spray. Bake 20 minutes or until fish flakes easily with a fork.

Makes 4 servings, 219 calories per serving

C-REEL RESULTS – Personal Food Diary

Name _____

Height _____ Weight _____

Date _____

Meal 1 – Time (AM) _____
_____
_____

Meal 2 – Time (AM) _____
_____
_____

Meal 3 – Time (PM) _____
_____
_____

Meal 4 – Time (PM) _____
_____
_____

Meal 5 – Time (PM) _____
_____
_____

Meal 6 – Time (PM) _____
_____
_____

C-REEL RESULTS – Personal Food Diary

Name _____

Height _____ Weight _____

Date _____

Meal 1 – Time (AM) _____
_____
_____

Meal 2 – Time (AM) _____
_____
_____

Meal 3 – Time (PM) _____
_____
_____

Meal 4 – Time (PM) _____
_____
_____

Meal 5 – Time (PM) _____
_____
_____

Meal 6 – Time (PM) _____
_____
_____

C-REEL RESULTS – Week 1-2 Explanation

This week, you will perform 15-20 minutes of cardio activity of your choice immediately before your workout. (treadmill walking, jogging, running, elliptical, stairmaster, etc.)

Complete the exercises in numerical order, straight down the list.

During each exercise, take three seconds on the way up, pause for one second, and take three seconds on the way down. That is one repetition (rep).

Begin with number 1 (Stability Ball Push-Up). Complete this exercise 6-8 times (6-8 reps), then rest for fifteen seconds before moving to number 2 (Stability Ball Push-Up). Continue until you finish with number 16 (cat stretch).

You will notice that each exercise is repeated. This means there are two sets of each exercise. Your total workout is 16 sets.

Complete this workout twice per week. Do not workout two days in a row. For example: workout on Monday and Thursday, or workout on Tuesday and Saturday.

See Week 1-2 exercise log to keep track of your progress.

Nutritional "Homework"

• **Drink 32 oz of water before 9am every morning**

Good Luck

Week 1-2 Fitness Log

Perform 15-20 minutes of cardio before workout

Excercise	Reps	Weight/Reps	Rest
1. Stability Ball Push-ups	6-8x	____/____	15 sec
2. Stability Ball Push-ups	6-8x	____/____	15 sec
3. Low Back Stretch	6-8x	____/____	15 sec
4. Low Back Stretch	6-8x	____/____	15 sec
5. Seated Forward Rear Delt Raise	6-8x	____/____	15 sec
6. Seated Forward Rear Delt Raise	6-8x	____/____	15 sec
7. Hip Thrust Stretch	6-8x	____/____	15 sec
8. Hip Thrust Stretch	6-8x	____/____	15 sec
9. Glute Lifts	6-8x	____/____	15 sec
10. Glute Lifts	6-8x	____/____	15 sec
11. Glute Stretch	6-8x	____/____	15 sec
12. Glute Stretch	6-8x	____/____	15 sec
13. One Arm Rows	6-8x	____/____	15 sec
14. One Arm Rows	6-8x	____/____	15 sec
15. Cat Stretch	6-8x	____/____	15 sec
16. Cat Stretch	6-8x	____/____	15 sec

C-REEL RESULTS – Week 3-4 Explanation

This week, you will perform 20-30 minutes of cardio activity of your choice immediately before your workout. (treadmill walking, jogging, running, elliptical, stairmaster, etc.)

Complete the exercises in numerical order, straight down the list.

During each exercise, take three seconds on the way up, pause for one second, and take three seconds on the way down. That is one repetition (rep).

Begin with number 1 (Stability Ball Push-Up). Complete this exercise 6-10 times (6-10 reps), then rest for fifteen seconds before moving to number 2 (Stability Ball Push-Up). Continue until you finish with number 24 (Partial Lateral Raises).

You will notice that each exercise is repeated. This means there are two sets of each exercise. Your total workout is 24 sets.

Complete this workout twice per week. Do not workout two days in a row. For example: workout on Monday and Thursday, or workout on Tuesday and Saturday.

See Week 3-4 exercise log to keep track of your progress.

Nutritional "Homework"

- **Drink 32 oz of water before 9am every morning**

- **Add another 32 oz of water between Noon and 3pm everyday**

- **Structure dinner, which should be meal No. 5 of the day (6 pm- 8pm). See *Dinner Options*.**

- **Do the best you can with the rest of the day.**

Good Luck

Week 3-4 Fitness Log

Perform 20-30 minutes of cardio before workout

Excercise	Reps	Weight/Reps	Rest
1. Stability Ball Push-ups	6-10	____/____	15 sec
2. Stability Ball Push-ups	6-10	____/____	15 sec
3. Low Back Stretch	6-10	____/____	15 sec
4. Low Back Stretch	6-10	____/____	15 sec
5. Towel Crunches	6-10	____/____	15 sec
6. Towel Crunches	6-10	____/____	15 sec
7. Seated Forward Rear Delt Raise	6-10	____/____	15 sec
8. Seated Forward Rear Delt Raise	6-10	____/____	15 sec
9. Hip Thrust Stretch	6-10	____/____	15 sec
10. Hip Thrust Stretch	6-10	____/____	15 sec
11. Squat Hold	30-60 second hold		15 sec
12. Squat Hold	30-60 second hold		15 sec
13. Glute Lifts	6-10	____/____	15 sec
14. Glute Lifts	6-10	____/____	15 sec
15. Glute Stretch	6-10	____/____	15 sec
16. Glute Stretch	6-10	____/____	15 sec
17. Butterfly Towel Crunches	6-10	____/____	15 sec
18. Butterfly Towel Crunches	6-10	____/____	15 sec
19. One Arm Rows	6-10	____/____	15 sec
20. One Arm Rows	6-10	____/____	15 sec
21. Cat Stretch	6-10	____/____	15 sec
22. Cat Stretch	6-10	____/____	15 sec
23. Partial Lateral Raises	6-10	____/____	15 sec
24. Partial Lateral Raises	6-10	____/____	15 sec

C-REEL RESULTS – Week 5-6 Explanation

This week, you will perform 30-40 minutes of cardio activity of your choice immediately before your workout. (treadmill walking, jogging, running, elliptical, stairmaster, etc.)

Complete the exercises in numerical order, straight down the list.

During each exercise, take three seconds on the way up, pause for one second, and take three seconds on the way down. That is one repetition (rep).

Begin with number 1 (Stability Ball Push-Up). Complete this exercise 6-12 times (6-12 reps), then do not rest before moving to number 2 (Low Back Stretch). Continue until you finish with number 16 (Modified Superman). Your total workout is 16 sets.

Complete this workout three times per week. Do not workout two days in a row. For example: workout on Monday, Wednesday and Friday, or workout on Tuesday, Thursday and Saturday.

See Week 5-6 exercise log to keep track of your progress.

Nutritional "Homework"

• **Consume 32oz of water before 9am every morning.**

• **Consume 32oz of water between Noon and 3pm everyday.**

• **Follow Dinner Options.**

• **Structure breakfast, which should be meal number 1 of the day (6am-8am). See –*Breakfast Options*.**

• **Do the best you can with the rest of the day.**

Good Luck

Week 5-6 Fitness Log

Perform 30-40 minutes of cardio before workout

Excercise	Reps	Weight/Reps	Rest
1. Stability Ball Push-ups	6-12	____/____	0 sec
2. Low Back Stretch	6-12	____/____	0 sec
3. Towel Crunches	6-12	____/____	0 sec
4. Kneeling DB Curls	6-12	____/____	0 sec
5. Seated Forward Rear Delt Raises	6-12	____/____	0 sec
6. Hip Thrust Stretch	6-12	____/____	0 sec
7. Squat Hold	30-60 second hold		0 sec
8. Tricep Kickbacks	6-12	____/____	0sec
9. Glute Lifts	6-12	____/____	0sec
10. Glute Stretch	6-12	____/____	0sec
11. Butterfly Towel Crunches	6-12	____/____	0 sec
12. Bridges	6-12	____/____	0 sec
13. One Arm Rows	6-12	____/____	0 sec
14. Cat Stretch	6-12	____/____	0 sec
15. Partial Lateral Raises	6-12	____/____	0 sec
16. Modified Superman	6-12	____/____	0 sec

C-REEL RESULTS – Week 7-8 Explanation

This week, you will warm-up for 5-10 minutes with a cardio activity of your choice immediately before your workout. (treadmill walking, jogging, running, elliptical, stairmaster, etc.)

Complete the exercises in numerical order, straight down the list.

During each exercise, take three seconds on the way up, pause for one second, and take three seconds on the way down. That is one repetition (rep).

Begin with number 1 (Kneeling DB Curls). Complete this exercise 10 times (10 reps), then rest for fifteen seconds before moving to number 2 (Kneeling DB Curls). Continue until you finish with number 16 (Partial Lateral Raise).

You will notice that each exercise is repeated. This means there are two sets of each exercise. Your total workout is 16 sets.

Complete this workout three times per week. Do not workout two days in a row. For example: workout on Monday, Wednesday and Friday, or workout on Tuesday, Thursday and Saturday.

Perform 15-20 minutes cardio activity of your choice immediately after your workout. (treadmill walking, jogging, running, elliptical, stairmaster, etc.)

See Week 7-8 exercise log to keep track of your progress.

Nutritional "Homework"

• **Consume 32oz of water before 9am every morning.**

• **Add 32 oz of water between 9am and Noon everyday.**

• **Consume 32oz of water between Noon and 3pm everyday.**

• **Follow *Dinner Options*.**

• **Follow *Breakfast Options*.**

• **Structure an afternoon snack, which should be meal number 4 of the day (3pm-5pm). See *Snack Options*.**

• **Do the best you can with the rest of the day.**

Good Luck

Week 7-8 Fitness Log

Warm-up: 5-10 minutes cardio before workout

Excercise	Reps	Weight/Reps	Rest
1. Kneeling DB Curls	10	____/____	15 sec
2. Kneeling DB Curls	10	____/____	15 sec
3. Towel Crunches	10	____/____	15 sec
4. Towel Crunches	10	____/____	15 sec
5. Tricep Kickbacks	10	____/____	15 sec
6. Tricep Kickbacks	10	____/____	15 sec
7. Squat Hold	30-60 second hold		15 sec
8. Squat Hold	30-60 second hold		15 sec
9. Bridges	10	____/____	15 sec
10. Bridges	10	____/____	15 sec
11. Butterfly Towel Crunches	10	____/____	15 sec
12. Butterfly Towel Crunches	10	____/____	15 sec
13. Modified Superman	10	____/____	15 sec
14. Modified Superman	10	____/____	15 sec
15. Partial Lateral Raises	10	____/____	15 sec
16. Partial Lateral Raises	10	____/____	15 sec

Perform 5-10 minutes cardio activity of your choice immediately after your workout

C-REEL RESULTS – Week 9-10 Explanation

This week, you will warm-up for 5-10 minutes with a cardio activity of your choice immediately before your workout. (treadmill walking, jogging, running, elliptical, stairmaster, etc.)

Complete the exercises in numerical order, straight down the list.

During each exercise, take three seconds on the way up, pause for one second, and take three seconds on the way down. That is one repetition (rep).

Begin with number 1 (Kneeling DB Curls). Complete this exercise 10-12 times (10-12 reps), then rest for twenty seconds before moving to number 2 (Kneeling DB Curls). Continue until you finish with number 24 (One Arm Rows).

You will notice that each exercise is repeated. This means there are two sets of each exercise. Your total workout is 24 sets.

Complete this workout three times per week. Do not workout two days in a row. For example: workout on Monday, Wednesday and Friday, or workout on Tuesday, Thursday and Saturday.

Perform 20-30 minutes cardio activity of your choice immediately after your workout. (treadmill walking, jogging, running, elliptical, stairmaster, etc.)

See Week 9-10 exercise log to keep track of your progress.

Nutritional "Homework"

- **Consume 32oz of water before 9am every morning.**

- **Add 32 oz of water between 9am and Noon everyday.**

- **Consume 32oz of water between Noon and 3pm everyday.**

- **Follow *Dinner Options*.**

- **Follow *Breakfast Options*.**

- **Follow *Snack Options* for afternoon snack.**

- **Structure morning snack, which should be meal number 2 of the day (9:30am-11am). See *Snack Options*.**

Good Luck

Week 9-10 Fitness Log

Warm-up: 5-10 minutes cardio before workout

Excercise	Reps	Weight/Reps	Rest
1. Kneeling DB Curls	10-12	____/____	20 sec
2. Kneeling DB Curls	10-12	____/____	20 sec
3. Towel Crunches	10-12	____/____	20 sec
4. Towel Crunches	10-12	____/____	20 sec
5. Stability Ball Push-ups	10-12	____/____	20 sec
6. Stability Ball Push-ups	10-12	____/____	20 sec
7. Tricep Kickbacks	10-12	____/____	20 sec
8. Tricep Kickbacks	10-12	____/____	20 sec
9. Squat Hold	30-60 second hold		20 sec
10. Squat Hold	30-60 second hold		20 sec
11. Seated Forward Rear Delt Raise	10-12	____/____	20 sec
12. Seated Forward Rear Delt Raise	10-12	____/____	20 sec
13. Bridges	10-12	____/____	20 sec
14. Bridges	10-12	____/____	20 sec
15. Butterfly Towel Crunches	10-12	____/____	20 sec
16. Butterfly Towel Crunches	10-12	____/____	20 sec
17. Glute Lifts	10-12	____/____	20 sec
18. Glute Lifts	10-12	____/____	20 sec
19. Modified Superman	10-12	____/____	20 sec
20. Modified Superman	10-12	____/____	20 sec
21. Partial Lateral Raises	10-12	____/____	20 sec
22. Partial Lateral Raises	10-12	____/____	20 sec
23. One Arm Rows	10-12	____/____	20 sec
24. One Arm Rows	10-12	____/____	20 sec

Perform 20-30 minutes cardio activity of your choice immediately after your workout

C-REEL RESULTS – Week 11-12 Explanation

This week, you will warm-up for 5-10 minutes with a cardio activity of your choice immediately before your workout. (treadmill walking, jogging, running, elliptical, stairmaster, etc.)

Complete the exercises in numerical order, straight down the list.

During each exercise, take three seconds on the way up, pause for one second, and take three seconds on the way down. That is one repetition (rep).

Begin with number 1 (Kneeling DB Curls). Complete this exercise 10-15 times (10-15 reps), then do not rest before moving to number 2 (Towel Crunches). Continue until you finish with number 16 (Cat Stretch). Your total workout is 16 sets.

Complete this workout three times per week. Do not workout two days in a row. For example: workout on Monday, Wednesday and Friday, or workout on Tuesday, Thursday and Saturday.

Perform 30-40 minutes cardio activity of your choice immediately after your workout. (treadmill walking, jogging, running, elliptical, stairmaster, etc.)

See Week 11-12 exercise log to keep track of your progress.

Nutritional "Homework"

- **Consume 32oz of water before 9am every morning.**

- **Add 32oz of water between 9am and Noon everyday.**

- **Drink 32oz of water between Noon and 3pm everyday.**

- **Follow *Dinner Options*.**

- **Follow *Breakfast Options*.**

- **Follow *Snack Options* for afternoon snack.**

- **Follow *Snack Options* for morning snack.**

- **Follow *Lunch Options*.**

- **Structure Lunch, which should be meal number 3 of the day (1pm-2pm). See Lunch Options.** Good Luck

Week 11-12 Fitness Log

Warm-up: 5-10 minutes cardio before workout

Excercise	Reps	Weight/Reps	Rest
1. Kneeling DB Curls	10-12	____/____	20 sec
2. Kneeling DB Curls	10-12	____/____	20 sec
3. Towel Crunches	10-12	____/____	20 sec
4. Towel Crunches	10-12	____/____	20 sec
5. Stability Ball Push-ups	10-12	____/____	20 sec
6. Stability Ball Push-ups	10-12	____/____	20 sec
7. Tricep Kickbacks	10-12	____/____	20 sec
8. Tricep Kickbacks	10-12	____/____	20 sec
9. Squat Hold	30-60 second hold		20 sec
10. Squat Hold	30-60 second hold		20 sec
11. Seated Forward Rear Delt Raise	10-12	____/____	20 sec
12. Seated Forward Rear Delt Raise	10-12	____/____	20 sec
13. Bridges	10-12	____/____	20 sec
14. Bridges	10-12	____/____	20 sec
15. Butterfly Towel Crunches	10-12	____/____	20 sec
16. Butterfly Towel Crunches	10-12	____/____	20 sec
17. Glute Lifts	10-12	____/____	20 sec
18. Glute Lifts	10-12	____/____	20 sec
19. Modified Superman	10-12	____/____	20 sec
20. Modified Superman	10-12	____/____	20 sec
21. Partial Lateral Raises	10-12	____/____	20 sec
22. Partial Lateral Raises	10-12	____/____	20 sec
23. One Arm Rows	10-12	____/____	20 sec
24. One Arm Rows	10-12	____/____	20 sec

Perform 30-40 minutes cardio activity of your choice immediately after your workout.

C-REEL RESULTS – Advanced Workout Log

This is an advanced workout for people with more than 3 years of weight training experience.

Monday and Thursday

Perform 10 minutes cardio to warm-up before workout:

Excercise	Reps	Weight/Reps	Weight/Reps
1. Incline Chest Press	15	____/____	____/____
2. Push-Ups	15	____/____	____/____
3. Chest Fly	15	____/____	____/____

Rest 30 seconds

4. Stationary Lunges	15	____/____	____/____
5. Leg Curls	15	____/____	____/____
6. Stationary Lunges	15	____/____	____/____
7. Leg Curls	15	____/____	____/____
8. Walking Lunges	15	____/____	____/____
9. 90° Low Back Extensions	15	____/____	____/____

Rest 30 seconds

10. Rear Delt Raises	15	____/____	____/____
11. Standing DB Shoulder Press	15	____/____	____/____
12. Rear Delt Raises	15	____/____	____/____
13. Standing Cable Curls	15	____/____	____/____
14. Standing DB Curls	15	____/____	____/____

Rest 30 seconds

15. Concentration Curls	15	____/____	____/____
16. 90° Low Back Extensions	15	____/____	____/____

Rest for 2 minutes and repeat once

Perform 20-30 minutes of cardio after Monday workout ONLY!

C-REEL RESULTS – Advanced Workout Log

This is an advanced workout for people with more than 3 years of weight training experience.

Wednesday and Saturday

Perform 10 minutes cardio to warm-up before workout:

Excercise	Reps	Weight/Reps	Weight/Reps
1. Bent Over DB Row	15	____/____	____/____
2. Lat Pulldowns	15	____/____	____/____
3. Bent Over DB Row	15	____/____	____/____

Rest 30 seconds

4. Stiff Leg Deadlifts	15	____/____	____/____
5. Leg Extensions	15	____/____	____/____
6. Stiff Leg Deadlifts	15	____/____	____/____
7. Leg Extensions	15	____/____	____/____
8. Abductor Machine	15	____/____	____/____
9. Ball Crunches with Weight	15	____/____	____/____

Rest 30 seconds

10. Upright Row	15	____/____	____/____
11. Reverse Lat Pulldowns	15	____/____	____/____
12. Upright Row	15	____/____	____/____
13. Bench Dip	15	____/____	____/____
14. Tricep Rope Pushdowns	15	____/____	____/____

Rest 30 seconds

15. Tricep Kickbacks	15	____/____	____/____
16. Ball Crunches with Weight	15	____/____	____/____

Rest for 2 minutes and repeat once

Perform 20-30 minutes of cardio after Saturday workout ONLY!

C-REEL RESULTS Exercises – Section A

Stability Ball Push-ups (Chest, Shoulder, Tricep muscles)

- To really make this exercise effective, it should take you 3 seconds to lower yourself down, pause, and then forcefully push yourself up.

- The farther you move out on the ball, the more difficult the exercise will become.

- At the finish position (the bottom) your head should be in front of your hands; and, your shoulders should be in line with your hands.

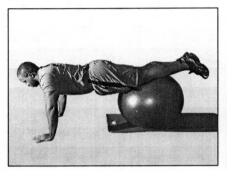 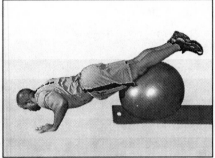

Low Back Stretch (Spinal Erectors)

- Hold stretch for 2 seconds and exhale, and then return feet back to the floor.

  Then repeat.

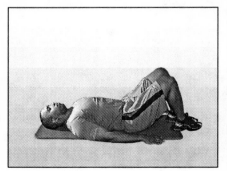 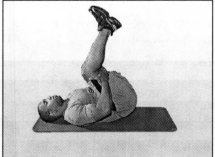

C-REEL RESULTS Exercises – Section A

Towel Crunch (Abs)

• Always push your head back into the towel at all times.

• Exhale and hold at the top for 3-4 seconds.

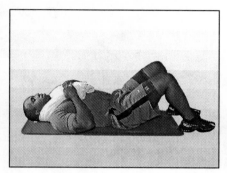 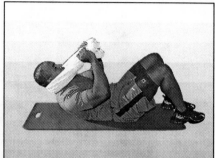

Kneeling Dumbbell Curls (Biceps)

• Keep your hips pushed forward.

• Keep your shoulders pinched together throughout the movement.
  Also, keep your shoulder blades back and down.

• Do not let your elbows move forward. Keep them back and stabilized.

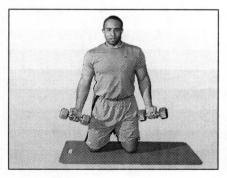 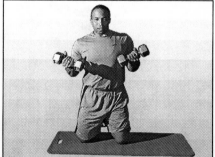

C-REEL RESULTS Exercises – Section B

Seated Forward Dumbbell Rear Delt Raises (Rear Shoulder Muscle)

- Keep your chest and head up at all times.

- Always keep a slight bend in your elbows from start to finish.

- Do not overly squeeze the dumbbells in your hands.

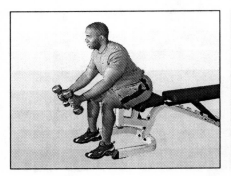 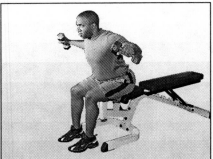

Hip Thrust Stretch (Hip Flexors)

- During the deepest part of the stretch, make sure your front knee is directly above your front ankle.

- As you move forward into the stretch, again keep your chest up.

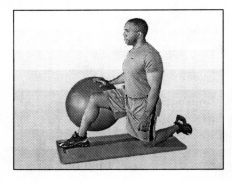 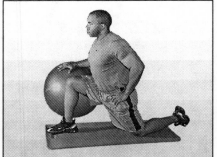

C-REEL RESULTS Exercises – Section B

30-60 second Squat Hold (Quads, Glutes)

- Slowly lower your body into the Squat position. It should take you 4-6 seconds to get into this position.

- Do not let your knee protrude too far beyond your toes in front.

  No pain in the knees.

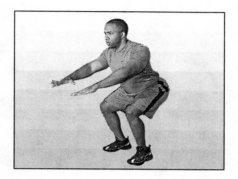

Tricep Kickbacks (Triceps)

- During the exercise, do not let your elbow move up and down. Stabilize your elbows to the sides of your body.

- Do not move too fast during the exercise. Pause for 2 seconds at the finish position.

- Pay close attention to my elbow. It does not move from start to finish

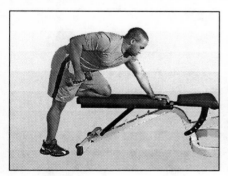 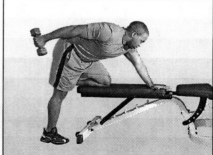

C-REEL RESULTS Exercises – Section C

Glute Lifts (Glutes, Hamstrings)

- Squeeze your hips up as far as you can comfortably.
  (or until hips are in line with shoulders)

- Push up from your heels.

- Slowly lower yourself down, but don't touch the floor. Keep your hamstrings
  and glutes tight from start to finish.

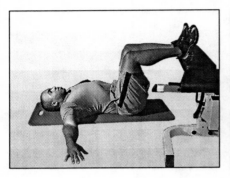 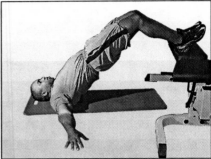

Glute Stretch (Glutes)

- Hold the stretch position for 2 seconds, release;
  and repeat 8-12 times on each side

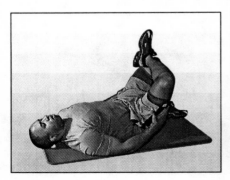 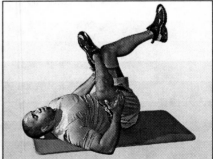

C-REEL RESULTS Exercises – Section C

Butterfly Towel Crunch (Lower, Upper Abs)

- Rest your head inside the towel. This is to help reduce strain on the neck.

- Exhale at the finish position.

- Squeeze your abs in that position for 3-5 seconds and return slowly to the starting position.

- Do not bounce up.

- Always keep your lower back pressed against the floor from start to finish.

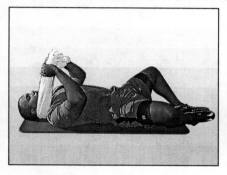 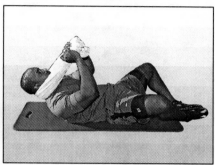

Bridges (Glutes, Hamstrings, Lower Back)

- Press your hips up towards the ceiling by pressing through the heels of your feet.

- When you lower your hips, do not touch the floor-keep your glutes and hamstrings under constant tension.

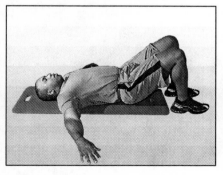 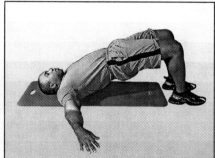

C-REEL RESULTS Exercises – Section D

One Arm Row (Upper Back Muscles)

- Use a "sawing" motion during this exercise.
- Keep your elbow close to your body.
- Do not squeeze the weights (dumbbells) too hard.

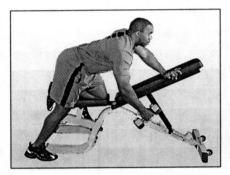 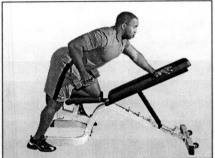

Cat Stretch (Low Back Stretch)

- Pull your bellybutton in towards your spine as your raise up.
- Inhale as your pull your bellybutton in.
- Exhale as you return to the starting position.

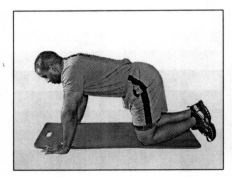 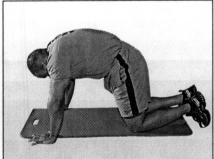

C-REEL RESULTS Exercises – Section D

Partial Lateral Raises (Side Shoulder Muscles)

- Do not squeeze the dumbbells too hard.

- Mentally concentrate on only using your shoulder muscles.

- Stand perfectly still during the exercise to help isolate your shoulder muscles even more.

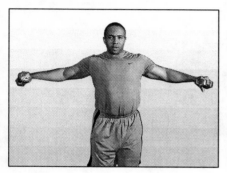 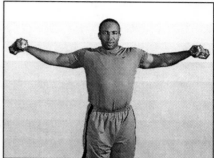

Modified Supermans (Low Back Muscles)

- Focus on just using your low back muscles during the exercise.

- You can leave your feet on the floor.

- If there is any low back pain-please skip this exercise.

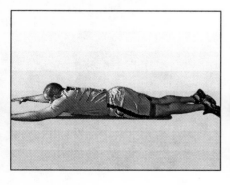 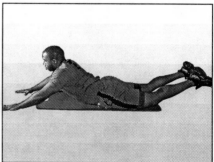

C-REEL RESULTS Exercises – Section E

Quadriceps Stretch (Front of Thigh Stretch)

- Make sure your right hand grabs your right ankle.

- Hold each stretch only 2 seconds then repeat 8-10 times.

- Make sure your knee always points towards the floor and not backwards.

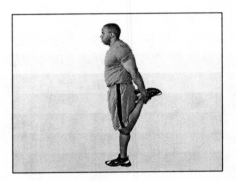

Hamstring Stretch (Back of Thigh Stretch)

- Please make sure your chest remains up, and your back is straight from start to finish.

- Hold the stretch for only 2 seconds, then repeat 8-10 times.

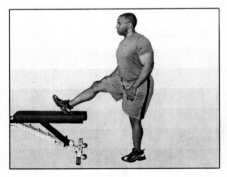 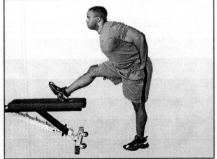

C-REEL RESULTS Exercises – Section E

Shoulder Stretch (Shoulder and Bicep Stretch)

- Make a fist and hold your arm up in line with your shoulder.

- Again, only hold the stretch for 2 seconds then repeat the stretch 8-10 times on each side.

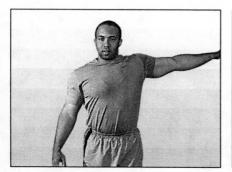 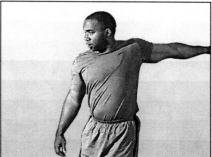

About the Author

John Henry Creel is a nationally-known personal trainer and coveted life-coach. His refreshing and revolutionary approach to physical fitness has achieved hundreds of body transformations for people of all ages, shapes, sizes and fitness levels. His direct approach to mental fitness has literally changed lives, sky-rocketing people's self esteem and making them more assertive, productive and motivated.

Men's Journal Magazine has repeatedly named John Henry Creel one of the Top 100 Trainers in the Nation. He's the official trainer of the NBA's *Cleveland Cavalier* Dance Team and has been featured on multiple national television and radio programs.

Creel is a former competitive natural body builder and has held the title of "Mr. Cincinnati". He has trained bodybuilders, figure competitors and Miss America Pageant contestants. But his true passion is EMPOWERING people just like you to make significant lifestyle changes through mind and body fitness.

Today Creel owns and operates Mind & Body Fitness, Inc., a personal training studio where he develops and implements customized fitness, strength-training and fat-loss nutritional programs for clients and members. He also operates JH Fitness & Consulting, Inc., which teaches and coaches other personal trainers and fitness center owners. Seeking to share the business of creating better minds and bodies, Creel spends much of his time conducting interactive seminars and creating informative lectures for groups both large and small.

Printed in the United States
89998LV00004B/37-210/A

9 781600 373176